Minimally Invasive Acute Care Surgery

Kosar A. Khwaja • Jose J. Diaz

Editors

Minimally Invasive Acute Care Surgery

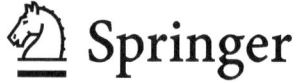 Springer

Editors
Kosar A. Khwaja, MD, MBA, MSc, FRCS, FACS
Director of Acute Care Surgery
Montreal General Hospital
Associate Director, Trauma Program
Departments of Surgery and Critical Care
McGill University Health Center
Montreal, QC, Canada

Jose J. Diaz, MD, CNS, FACS, FCCM
Chief Division of Acute Care Surgery
Acute Care Surgery
Fellowship, Program in Trauma
R Adams Cowley Shock Trauma Center
University of Maryland Medical Center
Baltimore, MD, USA

ISBN 978-3-319-64721-0   ISBN 978-3-319-64723-4   (eBook)
https://doi.org/10.1007/978-3-319-64723-4

Library of Congress Control Number: 2017959192

Printed on acid-free paper

This Springer imprint is published by Springer Nature
The registered company is Springer International Publishing AG
The registered company address is: Gewerbestrasse 11, 6330 Cham, Switzerland

I would like to dedicate this book to my beautiful wife, Amna, whose strength and perseverance never ceases to amaze me, and to my children, Noor, Zahra, and Leena, who inspire me on a daily basis to succeed in everything I do. I would like to thank my family, particularly my parents, who have always tried to support me in any way they can.

Furthermore, I would like to dedicate this book to my colleagues at the McGill University Health Centre who, despite facing important challenges, continue to advocate for their patients and deliver world-class patient care.

Kosar A. Khwaja, MD

I would like to dedicate this book to my wife, Dinah, and my children, Gabriella, Veronica, and Alejandro. They are my strength and inspiration while I care for the sickest patients in my community.

In addition, I want to dedicate this book to Raphael Chung, MD, who was my chairman of surgery during my residency at Huron Road Hospital/Cleveland Clinic Foundation Affiliate. He was my teacher, trusted mentor, and model academician who I came to emulate. Most of all, Dr. Chung was a maverick during the early era of laparoscopy asking how best to use the surgeon's newest tools. Yet, he would always be asking where was the evidence; if none, he would gather the evidence to demonstrate the idea had value.

Jose J. Diaz, MD

The main goal of this text is to ensure the safety of our surgical patients and to provide surgeons engaged in the practice of acute care surgery (ACS) additional guidance when considering the minimally invasive approach to emergency general surgery cases. This book bridges the gap between the minimally invasive surgery (MIS) expert who may not routinely be involved in the care of the acute care surgery patient and the ACS expert surgeon who may not have a routine MIS elective practice.

Since the early 1990s, with the addition of laparoscopy to the practice of general surgery, general surgeons have been pushing the envelope by introducing more minimally invasive surgical techniques in their elective surgical practice. As surgeons became more comfortable with the MIS approach, this approach was increasingly considered in the acute setting, leading to two observations:

1. Skilled MIS surgeons who had predominately an MIS elective practice were attempting similar techniques in the emergency general surgery population without the recognition of the severity and pathophysiology of the critically ill ACS patient and the physiologic effects of pneumoperitoneum in sick patients.
2. ACS surgeons who may not have a regular MIS elective practice were attempting minimally invasive approaches in high-risk emergency general surgery patients without having the expert MIS skill set.

The renewed scientific interest for acute surgical disease has resulted in the improved care of emergency general surgery patients. Patient selection, early recognition of severity of illness, shortened time to source control in sepsis, innovation in resuscitation and damage control, and postoperative management have all contributed to the improved outcomes for this patient population. In many institutions, trauma surgeons have taken the lead in the development of the acute care surgery program because of their expertise in the management of critically ill trauma and surgical intensive care patients. With the addition of emergency general surgery to a trauma and surgical intensive care practice, the acute care surgeon is now exposed to a more consistent operative experience.

It is important that MIS experts managing acute care surgery patients and ACS surgeons contemplating an MIS approach are well versed on the current indications, contraindications, and recommendations for the appropriate use of minimally invasive techniques in critically ill surgical patients. This book brings together the experts in MIS and the experts in ACS to outline a safe approach to managing acute care surgical diseases with an MIS approach.

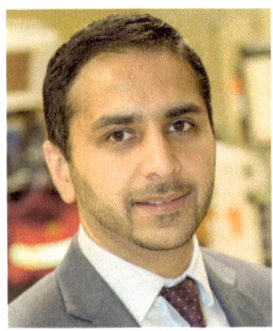

Kosar A. Khwaja, MD
Montreal, QC, Canada

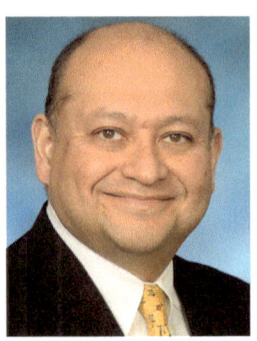

Jose J. Diaz, MD
Baltimore, MD, USA

Contents

1   Physiologic Effects of Pneumoperitoneum: Implications
    of Laparoscopy in Critically Ill Patients Undergoing Emergency
    Minimally Invasive Surgery 1
    Jeremy R. Grushka and Kosar A. Khwaja

2   Laparoscopic Exploration for Free Air 7
    Allison J. Tompeck and Mayur Narayan

3   Incarcerated Abdominal Wall Hernias: Tips and Tricks
    to the Minimally Invasive Approach 15
    Ciara R. Huntington and B. Todd Heniford

4   Laparoscopic Approach to the Acutely Incarcerated
    Paraesophageal Hernia 25
    Lee L. Swanström and Kristin Beard

5   Acute Care Surgery for Bariatric Surgery Emergencies 33
    Mark D. Kligman

6   Managing the Difficult Gallbladder in Acute Cholecystitis 45
    Chad G. Ball, Francis R. Sutherland, and S. Morad Hameed

7   Minimally Invasive Approach to Choledocholithiasis 53
    Caolan Walsh, Amy Neville, Diederick Jalink, and Fady K. Balaa

8   Laparoscopic Management of Perforated Ulcers 61
    Mohammed Hassan Al Mahroos and Liane S. Feldman

9   Minimally Invasive Strategies for the Treatment
    of Necrotizing Infected Pancreatitis: Video-Assisted
    Retroperitoneal Debridement (VARD) 67
    Jacques Mather and Jose J. Diaz

10 Laparoscopic Management of Small Bowel Obstruction 77
    John Hagen

11 Management of Appendicitis 81
    Benjamin Braslow

12 Minimally Invasive Approach to Acute Diverticulitis 89
    Matthew Randall Rosengart

13 Laparoscopic Re-exploration for Colorectal Surgery Complications 97
    Nathalie Wong-Chong and A. Sender Liberman

14 Minimally Invasive Approaches to Clostridium Difficile Colitis 107
Paul Waltz and Brian S. Zuckerbraun

15 Bedside Laparoscopy in the Intensive Care Unit........................... 115
Bradley W. Thomas and Ronald F. Sing

16 Laparoscopic Exploration for Trauma..................................... 119
Zachary Englert and Jose J. Diaz

Index 127

Contributors

Fady K. Balaa, MD, BSc, MD, MMed, FRCSC The Ottawa Hospital, General Campus, Ottawa, ON, Canada

Chad G. Ball, MD, MSC, FRCSC, FACS Foothills Medical Center, Department of Surgery, Calgary, Alberta, Canada

Kristin Beard, MD Portland Providence Hospital, Providence Cancer Center, Portland, OR, USA

Benjamin Braslow, MD PENN Presbyterian Medical Center, Division of Trauma, Surgical Critical and Emergency Surgery, Philadelphia, PA, USA

Jose J. Diaz, MD, CNS, FACS, FCCM R Adams Cowley Shock Trauma Center, University of Maryland School of Medicine, Baltimore, MD, USA

Zachary Englert, DO R Adams Cowley Shock Trauma Center, University of Maryland School of Medicine, Baltimore, MD, USA

Liane S. Feldman, MD, FACS, FRCS Steinberg-Bernstein Centre for Minimally Invasive Surgery and Innovation, Division of General Surgery, McGill University Health Centre, Montreal, QC, Canada

Jeremy R. Grushka, MD, MSc, FRCSC McGill University Health Center, Division of General and Trauma Surgery, Department of Critical Care Medicine, Montreal General Hospital, Montreal, QC, Canada

John Hagen, MD, FRCS(C) Department of Surgery University of Toronto, Humber River Hospital, Toronto, ON, Canada

S. Morad Hameed, MD, MPH, FRCSC, FACS Vancouver General Hospital, Department of Trauma, Vancouver, BC, Canada

B. Todd Heniford, MD, FACS Division of Gastrointestinal and Minimally Invasive Surgery, Carolinas Medical Center, Department of Surgery, Charlotte, NC, USA

Ciara R. Huntington, MD Carolinas Medical Center, Department of Surgery, Charlotte, NC, USA

Diederick Jalink, MD, FRCS Kingston Health Sciences Centre, Department of General Surgery, Kingston, ON, Canada

Kosar A. Khwaja, MD, MBA, MSc, FRCS, FACS McGIll University Health Centre, McGill University, Departments of Surgery and Critical Care, Montreal, QC, Canada

Mark D. Kligman, MD Department of Surgery, Center for Weight Management & Wellness, University of Maryland, School of Medicine, Baltimore, MD, USA

A. Sender Liberman, MD, BSc, MD, FRCSC, FACS, FASCRS McGill University Health Centre, Department of Colon & Rectal Surgery, Montreal, QC, Canada

Mohammed Hassan Al Mahroos, MD, FRCSC McGill University Health Centre, Department of Surgery, Montreal, QC, Canada

Jacques Mather, MD, MPH R Adams Cowley Shock Trauma Center, University of Maryland School of Medicine, Baltimore, MD, USA

Mayur Narayan, MD, MPH, MBA, FACS, FCCM, FICS University of Texas Southwestern Medical Center, Department of Surgery, Dallas, TX, USA

Amy Neville, MD, MSc The Ottawa Hospital, University of Ottawa, Department of Surgery, Ottawa, ON, Canada

Matthew Randall Rosengart, MD, MPH University of Pittsburgh Medical Center, Department of Surgery, Pittsburgh, PA, USA

Ronald F. Sing, DO, FACS The F.H. "Sammy" Ross Jr Trauma Center, Department of Surgery, Carolinas Medical Center, Charlotte, NC, USA

Francis R. Sutherland, MD, FRCSC Foothills Medical Center, Department of Surgery, Calgary, AB, Canada

Lee L. Swanström, MD Oregon Health and Sciences University, Portland, OR, USA

IHU-Strasbourg, Strasbourg, France

Bradley W. Thomas, MD, FACS Division of Acute Care Surgery, Department of Surgery, Carolinas Medical Center, Charlotte, NC, USA

Allison J. Tompeck, MD University of Texas Southwestern Medical Center, Department of Surgery, Dallas, TX, USA

Caolan Walsh, MD, FRCSC The Ottawa Hospital, Department of General Surgery, Ottawa, ON, Canada

Paul Waltz, MD University of Pittsburgh Medical Center, Department of Surgery, Pittsburgh, PA, USA

Nathalie Wong-Chong, BHSc, MD McGill University Health Centre, Department of General Surgery, Montreal, QC, Canada

Brian S. Zuckerbraun, MD, FACS University of Pittsburgh Medical Center, VA Pittsburgh Healthcare System, Pittsburgh, PA, USA

Physiologic Effects of Pneumoperitoneum: Implications of Laparoscopy in Critically Ill Patients Undergoing Emergency Minimally Invasive Surgery

Jeremy R. Grushka and Kosar A. Khwaja

Over the past 30 years, minimally invasive surgery (MIS) has revolutionized the practice of modern surgery and has become standard for the treatment of many surgical conditions. Multiple benefits of MIS compared to traditional open surgery are well documented including less induced surgical trauma and physiologic stress, reduced in-hospital length of stay, decreased postoperative pain, and faster functional recovery as well as improved cosmesis [1–4]. Decades of research examining the physiologic changes, clinical outcomes, and complications associated with MIS, along with major technological advances in optics and MIS instrumentation and surgical training, have led to near universal acceptance of MIS in all surgical specialties for both advanced elective and select emergency operations. For the acute care surgery (ACS) patient, MIS provides clear visualization of the thoracic cavity, the peritoneal space, and the anterior abdominal wall and, unlike other diagnostic modalities, has the potential benefit for therapeutic intervention while also decreasing rates of unnecessary nontherapeutic procedures. Despite these clear potential advantages, MIS has yet to achieve widespread acceptance within the ACS community. Debate continues to surround both the appropriate indications and applications of MIS in the acute emergency general surgery patient.

Laparoscopy requires the insufflation of carbon dioxide (CO_2) into the abdominal cavity in order to allow for surgical exposure and maintain operative freedom. The working space created by CO_2 pneumoperitoneum is dependent on the pressure of the gas presented to the patient. The resulting increased intra-abdominal pressure can induce many pathophysiologic disturbances that may increase the risk of perioperative complications due to the hemodynamic and cardiorespiratory changes caused by the pneumoperitoneum. While patients who are otherwise healthy will tolerate laparoscopy well, patients who require emergency surgical interventions are often displaying abnormal physiology due to underlying medical comorbidities, advanced age, or critical illness. Therefore, a thorough understanding of the physiologic changes caused by the pneumoperitoneum in emergency surgical patients undergoing laparoscopic surgery is needed to ensure optimal perioperative support and outcome for these patients.

Physiologic Changes

After an extensive literature review of both animal and human studies, O'Malley and Cunningham provide an excellent overview of the cardiovascular response (Table 1.1) and regional circulatory changes (Table 1.2) associated with pneumoperitoneum [5].

Respiratory Changes

CO_2 is the gas of choice for establishing pneumoperitoneum during laparoscopic surgery because it is noncombustible, extremely soluble, and readily eliminated by the lungs [6]. Despite the proven effectiveness and protection of CO_2 for insufflation in laparoscopy, the physiology of the respiratory system is affected by pneumoperitoneum. With insufflation, the increase in intra-abdominal pressure impairs excursion of the diaphragm and leads to compression of the lower lobes, reducing the total volume of the lungs. As a result, both a substantial decrease in pulmonary compliance and increase in maximum respiratory resistance are seen with

J.R. Grushka
McGill University Health Center, Division of General and Trauma Surgery, Department of Critical Care Medicine, Montreal General Hospital, Montreal, Quebec, Canada
e-mail: jeremy.grushka@mcgill.ca

K.A. Khwaja (✉)
Acute Care Surgery, MGH, Trauma Program, Critical Care Medicine, McGIll University Health Centre, McGill University, Departments of Surgery and Critical Care, Montreal, Quebec, Canada
e-mail: Kosar.Khwaja@mcgill.ca

© Springer International Publishing AG 2018
K.A. Khwaja, J.J. Diaz (eds.), *Minimally Invasive Acute Care Surgery*, https://doi.org/10.1007/978-3-319-64723-4_1

Table 1.1 Cardiovascular response associated with pneumoperitoneum

Measurement method	MAP	SVR	HR	PCWP	CVP	CI/CO
TEE	↑	↑	↔		↑	↓
ED	↑	↑	↔			↓
TEE	↑		↑			↓
TBC	↑	↑	↔			↔
PAC	↑	↑			↑	↑
PAC	↑	↑	↔	↑	↑	↓
PAC	↑		↔	↑	↑	↓
PAC	↑		↔	↑	↑	↓
TBC	↔	↑	↔	↓		
PAC	↑	↑	↔	↑		↓
ED	↑		↔			↓
TBC	↑			↑		↓
PAC	↑	↑				↓
PAC	↑	↑				↓
TBC	↔	↑	↔			↓
PAC	↑	↑	↔			↓

MAP mean arterial blood pressure; *SVR* systemic vascular resistance; *HR* heart rate; *CVP* central venous pressure; *PCWP* pulmonary capillary wedge pressure; *CI/CO* cardiac index/cardiac output; *PAC* pulmonary artery catheter; *ED* esophageal Doppler; *TEE* transesophageal echocardiography; *TBC* transthoracic bioimpedance ↑ increase, ↓ decrease, ↔ no change

Table 1.2 Regional circulatory changes associated with pneumoperitoneum

Region	Circulatory changes
Brain	↑ cerebral blood flow ↑ intracranial pressure ↔ cerebral perfusion pressure
Liver	↔ hepatic artery blood flow ↓ portal vein blood flow ↓ hepatic vein blood flow ↓ total hepatic blood flow ↓ hepatic microcirculation
Bowel	↓ gastric pHi ↓ gastric, duodenal, jejunal, colonic microcirculation ↓ superior mesenteric artery flow
Kidney	↓ renal artery blood flow ↓ renal vein blood flow ↓ renal cortical perfusion ↓ renal medullary perfusion
Lower limbs	↓ femoral vein blood flow

H human; *A* animal; ↓ decrease; ↑ increase; ↔ no change

establishing CO_2 pneumoperitoneum [7–9]. Physiologically, this is manifested as a decrease in functional residual capacity, with an increase in alveolar dead space and resultant ventilation/perfusion (V/Q) mismatch [10]. This is further compounded by changes in patient position as required to complete the surgical procedure, including Trendelenburg and reverse Trendelenburg positions. Though rarely clinically significant in healthy patients, the relative hypoxemia resulting from V/Q mismatch and pulmonary shunting may

be of paramount importance in a critically ill patient undergoing emergency surgery [11].

Carbon dioxide is insufflated into the peritoneal cavity at a rate of 4–6 L/min to a pressure of 10–20 mmHg. The pressure is maintained by a constant gas flow of 200–400 ml/min. An extremely soluble gas, CO_2, is readily absorbed through the peritoneal cavity into the systemic circulation leading to respiratory acidosis by the generation of carbonic acid. In patients with normal pulmonary function and host physiology, this respiratory acidosis is typically not clinically significant. However, patients with severe cardiopulmonary disease or acute critical illness, such as sepsis, are at increased risk for developing profound hypercarbia and acidemia during CO_2 pneumoperitoneum [12]. Patients presenting with significant metabolic acidosis secondary to sepsis should *not* undergo CO_2 pneumoperitoneum because of the risk of further profound acidemia that can ensue. All patients undergoing laparoscopic surgery warrant close monitoring of their cardiorespiratory parameters ensuring adequate CO_2 clearance through ventilation.

It is important to note that data from elective procedures have shown that major physiologic benefits of laparoscopy versus the open technique are realized postoperatively, specifically relating to lung mechanics. There is a smaller reduction in FRC, FEV1, FRC, and compliance postoperatively in the patients undergoing a laparoscopic approach versus open. Furthermore, there is less severe pulmonary atelectasis in this group as well. Finally, the laparoscopic group tends to mobilize earlier which can contribute to a return to normal lung mechanics and may decrease postoperative complications such as deep vein thrombosis and pulmonary embolism. It is unclear to what extent, if any, are these benefits realized in patients who have been admitted to the ICU *pre*operatively with prolonged intubation, on higher PEEP and FiO_2 with already V/Q mismatch.

Cardiovascular Changes

Cardiovascular system effects during CO_2 pneumoperitoneum include an increase in systemic vascular resistance, mean arterial blood pressure, and myocardial filling pressures and a decrease in cardiac output, with little change in heart rate [7, 11, 13–16]. These physiologic changes are dependent on multiple variables including intra-abdominal pressure, patient position, CO_2 absorption, and duration of the procedure. A euvolemic preoperative intravascular volume status is essential to avoid cardiovascular depression secondary to decreased preload during laparoscopic surgery [17]. While initial insufflation of the peritoneal cavity results in a transient increase in cardiac preload, a steady state of decreased blood circulation within the inferior vena cava comes after due to the compressive effects of continued intra-abdominal pressure leading to decreased stroke volume and increased heart rate in order to maintain a constant cardiac output [12].

Hypercarbia has direct and indirect sympathoadrenal stimulating effects on cardiovascular functions. Mild levels of hypercarbia ($PaCO_2$ 45–50 mmHg) rarely produce clinically significant cardiovascular effects, while moderate to severe levels of hypercarbia can produce clinically significant cardiovascular events due to myocardial depression and pulmonary vasodilation [18]. The critically ill patient requiring emergency surgery typically demonstrates abnormal physiology and has impaired ventilator capacity to eliminate this increased CO_2 load [19]. The exact etiology of the hemodynamic changes during laparoscopy in the septic state is undetermined. It remains unclear whether these changes are due to a direct myocardial inhibitory effect of the acidosis or are secondary to decreased venous return and increased afterload created by the intraperitoneal pressure. Both factors are potentially contributory. In general, increased intra-abdominal pressure (up to 12–15 mmHg) decreases venous return, which results in reduced preload and cardiac output, without adequate intravascular volume loading [15]. Put together, laparoscopic intervention, when used in septic patients, should be used with caution.

Renal Changes

Oliguria is the most common renal effect of pneumoperitoneum [20–22]. Increased intra-abdominal pressure may lead to diminished renal function due to compression of renal parenchyma and renal vessels. At an intra-abdominal pressure of 20 mmHg, renal cortical blood flow is reduced by 60–75% that returns to normal after desufflation [23, 24]. The decrease in renal blood flow and cortical and medullary perfusion observed during pneumoperitoneum causes a reduction in glomerular filtration rate (GFR), urinary output, and creatinine clearance [22, 25–27]. Despite this drop, however, there are no long-term renal sequelae, even in patients with pre-existing renal disease, and pneumoperitoneum-induced renal failure does not occur. The exact mechanism of renal blood flow disturbance by pneumoperitoneum is still to be concluded although volume status may play a major role.

Additionally, the release of neurohumoral factors in response to the increased intra-abdominal pressure further alters renal function. During laparoscopy, the decreased renal perfusion secondary to increased intra-abdominal pressure activates the renin-angiotensin-aldosterone system resulting in renal cortical vasoconstriction. Serum levels of ADH, renin, and aldosterone are significantly increased during laparoscopic procedures [28].

Immunologic Changes

According to Karantonis' review, studies report that the laparoscopic approach is associated with a lower rise of inflammatory markers such as cortisol, CRP, TNF alpha, and IL-6 compared to laparotomy. Furthermore, in a peritonitis model, researchers have shown that macrophages after laparoscopy display a higher basal immune performance. The acute phase inflammatory response associated with perioperative sepsis was shown to be relatively attenuated during laparoscopy in contrast to laparotomy. Thereafter, the immune function seems to be preserved in a more efficient manner following laparoscopy [29]. Although these findings are intriguing, it is difficult at this time to assess the clinical importance and should not be used in the decision-making process when deciding open laparotomy versus a laparoscopic approach for an acute care surgery patient with intra-abdominal sepsis.

Physiologic Complications of Pneumoperitoneum for the Acute Care Surgery Patient

Cardiac arrhythmias are often transient and of little clinical significance with ventricular ectopic beats being the most common. Reflex vagal stimulation and peritoneal irritation from rapid insufflation of the peritoneal cavity during the initiation of pneumoperitoneum may cause nodal arrhythmias, bradyarrhythmias, or cardiac arrest [30]. Arrhythmias can also be reduced if CO_2 is insufflated at a rate of <1 L/min and $PaCO_2$ is maintained within normal range by mechanically increasing the minute ventilation [31].

Pneumothorax develops in 0.03% of cases as a result of leakage through vulnerable points in the diaphragm and typically do not require treatment but may require tube thoracostomy if it is under tension or interferes with ventilation or oxygenation [32]. A sudden increase in peak airway pressures, end-tidal CO_2, or arterial desaturation during laparoscopy is highly suggestive of an acquired tension pneumothorax, and a tube thoracostomy should be performed. If it is unclear which side may have the tension pneumothorax, bilateral decompression may be needed after immediate cessation of CO_2 insufflation and opening of all port air valves.

Venous gas embolism is a rare but potentially fatal complication. It may occur if air or carbon dioxide is insufflated directly into a blood vessel or by gas being drawn into a vessel by the Venturi effect. The physiological effects of venous gas embolism are more drastic with air compared with CO_2 due to its decreased blood solubility. Early clinical signs of venous gas embolism include acute hypotension, desaturation, and "mill wheel" murmur [33]. Complete hemodynamic collapse can rapidly follow the onset of clinical symptoms unless rapidly acted upon. Prompt treatment of venous gas embolism includes immediate discontinuation of gas insufflation, placement of the patient in left lateral decubitus position, and the gas aspirated via a central line.

Challenges of Laparoscopy in Emergency General Surgery

Emergency general surgery represents 11% of surgical admissions and 50% of surgical mortality in the United States [34]. Emergency general surgery encompasses the care of the most acutely ill, highest-risk, and most costly general surgery patients [35–37]. Patients undergoing emergency general surgery are up to 8 times more likely to die postoperatively compared to patients undergoing the same surgical procedure electively [36]. The perioperative complication rate in this population is greater than 50%, and up to 15% of patients will be readmitted to hospital within 30 days of hospital discharge [34–36, 38]. Patients requiring emergency general surgery procedures often present to hospital with significant comorbidities and physiologic derangements including hypovolemia, lactic acidosis, hypercarbia, and distributive or hemorrhagic shock. Most published evidence maintains hemodynamic instability to be an absolute contraindication to laparoscopy in emergency general surgery, and currently laparoscopy has no role in hemodynamically unstable patients [39]. While a large number of laparoscopic surgeries are performed each year, there are several non-negligible pathophysiologic changes that occur during pneumoperitoneum that may increase the potential morbidity of acute care surgical patients requiring emergency surgery. As the complexity of the laparoscopic operation increases, longer time duration of CO_2 insufflation and elevated intra-abdominal pressure is required, further magnifying physiologic alterations in emergency general surgery patients. Sound clinical judgment is needed to decide whether or not the benefits of a laparoscopic procedure outweigh the potential benefits for the patient in question.

Conclusion

Minimally invasive surgical techniques are continuously evolving but remain limited in acute care surgery. Current evidence supports the utility of laparoscopy as both diagnostic and therapeutic tool in select groups of hemodynamically normal patients requiring emergency general surgery. Hemodynamic instability remains an absolute contraindication to laparoscopy in acute care surgery. Patients requiring emergency general surgery often present with abnormal

physiology, advanced disease, and signs of clinical shock, and the added physiologic burden of pneumoperitoneum and potentially longer operative time may not outweigh the known benefits of laparoscopy seen in the elective setting. Significant respiratory, cardiac, and renal physiologic changes occur with increased intra-abdominal pressure secondary to CO_2 pneumoperitoneum, and these changes may not be appropriate for a critically ill patient requiring emergency surgery.

Take-Home Messages

The acute care surgeon must recall the following when deciding whether or not to perform an emergency operation via an open or closed technique:

• There are several non-negligible pathophysiologic changes that occur during pneumoperitoneum.
• With excellent understanding of the factors causing alterations in physiology, many measures can be undertaken to prevent complications that sometimes can prove to be fatal.
• Low intra-abdominal pressures during laparoscopic surgery should be encouraged to minimize the potential for numerous complications.

Key References

1. Barkun JS, Barkun AN, Sampalis JS, Fried G, Taylor B, Wexler MJ, Goresky CA, Meakins JL. Randomised controlled trial of laparoscopic versus mini cholecystectomy. The McGill Gallstone Treatment Group. Lancet. 1992;340(8828):1116–9.
2. Epstein AJ, Groeneveld PW, Harhay MO, Yang F, Polsky D. Impact of minimally invasive surgery on medical spending and employee absenteeism. JAMA Surg. 2013;148(7):641–7.
3. Jones DB, Soper NJ. Laparoscopic general surgery: current status and future potential. AJR Am J Roentgenol. 1994;163(6):1295–301.
4. Soper NJ, Brunt LM, Kerbl K. Laparoscopic general surgery. N Engl J Med. 1994;330(6):409–19.
5. O'Malley C, Cunningham AJ. Physiologic changes during laparoscopy. Anesthesiol Clin North Am. 2001;19(1):1–19.
6. Seed RF, Shakespeare TF, Muldoon MJ. Carbon dioxide homeostasis during anaesthesia for laparoscopy. Anaesthesia. 1970;25(2):223–31.
7. Makinen MT, Yli-Hankala A. The effect of laparoscopic cholecystectomy on respiratory compliance as determined by continuous spirometry. J Clin Anesth. 1996;8(2):119–22.
8. Pelosi P, Foti G, Cereda M, Vicardi P, Gattinoni L. Effects of carbon dioxide insufflation for laparoscopic cholecystectomy on the respiratory system. Anaesthesia. 1996;51(8):744–9.
9. Rauh R, Hemmerling TM, Rist M, Jacobi KE. Influence of pneumoperitoneum and patient positioning on respiratory system compliance. J Clin Anesth. 2001;13(5):361–5.
10. Puri GD, Singh H. Ventilatory effects of laparoscopy under general anaesthesia. Br J Anaesth. 1992;68(2):211–3.

11. Haydon GH, Dillon J, Simpson KJ, Thomas H, Hayes PC. Hypoxemia during diagnostic laparoscopy: a prospective study. Gastrointest Endosc. 1996;44(2):124–8.

12. Wittgen CM, Andrus CH, Fitzgerald SD, Baudendistel LJ, Dahms TE, Kaminski DL. Analysis of the hemodynamic and ventilatory effects of laparoscopic cholecystectomy. Arch Surg. 1991;126(8):997–1000. discussion −1.

13. Ninomiya K, Kitano S, Yoshida T, Bandoh T, Baatar D, Matsumoto T. Comparison of pneumoperitoneum and abdominal wall lifting as to hemodynamics and surgical stress response during laparoscopic cholecystectomy. Surg Endosc. 1998;12(2):124–8.

14. McLaughlin JG, Scheeres DE, Dean RJ, Bonnell BW. The adverse hemodynamic effects of laparoscopic cholecystectomy. Surg Endosc. 1995;9(2):121–4.

15. Joris JL, Chiche JD, Canivet JL, Jacquet NJ, Legros JJ, Lamy ML. Hemodynamic changes induced by laparoscopy and their endocrine correlates: effects of clonidine. J Am Coll Cardiol. 1998;32(5):1389–96.

16. Haxby EJ, Gray MR, Rodriguez C, Nott D, Springall M, Mythen M. Assessment of cardiovascular changes during laparoscopic hernia repair using oesophageal Doppler. Br J Anaesth. 1997;78(5):515–9.

17. Ho HS, Gunther RA, Wolfe BM. Intraperitoneal carbon dioxide insufflation and cardiopulmonary functions. Laparoscopic cholecystectomy in pigs. Arch Surg. 1992;127(8):928–32. discussion 32–3

18. Rasmussen JP, Dauchot PJ, DePalma RG, Sorensen B, Regula G, Anton AH, Gravenstein JS. Cardiac function and hypercarbia. Arch Surg. 1978;113(10):1196–200.

19. Greif WM, Forse RA. Hemodynamic effects of the laparoscopic pneumoperitoneum during sepsis in a porcine endotoxic shock model. Ann Surg. 1998;227(4):474–80.

20. Nishio S, Takeda H, Yokoyama M. Changes in urinary output during laparoscopic adrenalectomy. BJU Int. 1999;83(9):944–7.

21. Nguyen NT, Perez RV, Fleming N, Rivers R, Wolfe BM. Effect of prolonged pneumoperitoneum on intraoperative urine output during laparoscopic gastric bypass. J Am Coll Surg. 2002;195(4):476–83.

22. McDougall EM, Monk TG, Wolf JS Jr, Hicks M, Clayman RV, Gardner S, Humphrey PA, Sharp T, Martin K. The effect of prolonged pneumoperitoneum on renal function in an animal model. J Am Coll Surg. 1996;182(4):317–28.

23. Shuto K, Kitano S, Yoshida T, Bandoh T, Mitarai Y, Kobayashi M. Hemodynamic and arterial blood gas changes during carbon dioxide and helium pneumoperitoneum in pigs. Surg Endosc. 1995;9(11):1173–8.

24. Chiu AW, Chang LS, Birkett DH, Babayan RK. The impact of pneumoperitoneum, pneumoretroperitoneum, and gasless laparoscopy on the systemic and renal hemodynamics. J Am Coll Surg. 1995;181(5):397–406.

25. Koivusalo AM, Kellokumpu I, Ristkari S, Lindgren L. Splanchnic and renal deterioration during and after laparoscopic cholecystectomy: a comparison of the carbon dioxide pneumoperitoneum and the abdominal wall lift method. Anesth Analg. 1997;85(4):886–91.

26. Hamilton BD, Chow GK, Inman SR, Stowe NT, Winfield HN. Increased intra-abdominal pressure during pneumoperitoneum stimulates endothelin release in a canine model. J Endourol. 1998;12(2):193–7.

27. Dolgor B, Kitano S, Yoshida T, Bandoh T, Ninomiya K, Matsumoto T. Vasopressin antagonist improves renal function in a rat model of pneumoperitoneum. J Surg Res. 1998;79(2):109–14.

28. Ortega AE, Peters JH, Incarbone R, Estrada L, Ehsan A, Kwan Y, Spencer CJ, Moore-Jeffries E, Kuchta K, Nicoloff JT. A prospective randomized comparison of the metabolic and stress hormonal responses of laparoscopic and open cholecystectomy. J Am Coll Surg. 1996;183(3):249–56.

29. Karantonis FF, Nikiteas N, Perrea D, Vlachou A, Giamarellos-Bourboulis EJ, Tsigris C, Kostakis A. Evaluation of the effects of laparotomy and laparoscopy on the immune system in intra-abdominal sepsis--a review. J Investig Surg. 2008;21(6):330–9.

30. Shifren JL, Adlestein L, Finkler NJ. Asystolic cardiac arrest: a rare complication of laparoscopy. Obstet Gynecol. 1992;79(5 (Pt 2)):840–1.

31. Crist DW, Gadacz TR. Complications of laparoscopic surgery. Surg Clin North Am. 1993;73(2):265–89.

32. Glauser FL, Bartlett RH. Pneumoperitoneum in association with pneumothorax. Chest. 1974;66(5):536–40.

33. Deziel DJ, Millikan KW, Economou SG, Doolas A, Ko ST, Airan MC. Complications of laparoscopic cholecystectomy: a national survey of 4,292 hospitals and an analysis of 77,604 cases. Am J Surg. 1993;165(1):9–14.

34. Scott JW, Olufajo OA, Brat GA, Rose JA, Zogg CK, Haider AH, Salim A, Havens JM. Use of National Burden to define operative emergency general surgery. JAMA Surg. 2016;151(6):e160480.

35. Kassin MT, Owen RM, Perez SD, Leeds I, Cox JC, Schnier K, Sadiraj V, Sweeney JF. Risk factors for 30-day hospital readmission among general surgery patients. J Am Coll Surg. 2012;215(3):322–30.

36. Havens JM, Peetz AB, Do WS, Cooper Z, Kelly E, Askari R, Reznor G, Salim A. The excess morbidity and mortality of emergency general surgery. J Trauma Acute Care Surg. 2015;78(2):306–11.

37. Gale SC, Shafi S, Dombrovskiy VY, Arumugam D, Crystal JS. The public health burden of emergency general surgery in the United States: a 10-year analysis of the Nationwide inpatient sample–2001 to 2010. J Trauma Acute Care Surg. 2014;77(2):202–8.

38. Kwan TL, Lai F, Lam CM, Yuen WC, Wai A, Siu YC, Shung E, Law WL. Population-based information on emergency colorectal surgery and evaluation on effect of operative volume on mortality. World J Surg. 2008;32(9):2077–82.

39. Ball CG, Karmali S, Rajani RR. Laparoscopy in trauma: an evolution in progress. Injury. 2009;40(1):7–10.

Allison J. Tompeck and Mayur Narayan

Introduction/Rationale

Laparoscopic exploration is a minimally invasive approach for the investigation and potential intervention of pneumoperitoneum or intra-abdominal free air. The procedure entails examination of the intra-abdominal organs, retroperitoneal surfaces, peritoneal lining, and free peritoneal fluid. Adjuncts, such as intraoperative esophagogastroduodenoscopy (EGD), methylene blue, and Pinpoint™ (Novadaq, Bonita Springs, FL) permit visualization of hollow organs, identify occult injury, and map the mesenteric vasculature.

The morbidity associated with a laparotomy incision ranges from 5% to 22% [1]. Conversely, laparoscopy consistently endorses improvements in numerous postoperative outcome measures. These include decreased length of stay, reduced rate of postoperative complications such as surgical site infections, decreased postoperative pain, and overall faster recovery with an expedited return to work [2, 3]. Long-term advantages are fewer intra-abdominal adhesions and a reduced rate of incisional hernia formation. Therefore, laparoscopy is the contemporary mainstay for surgical management of gallbladder disease, appendicitis, staging of intra-abdominal malignancy, and gynecologic pathology [1, 4, 5]. In the acute care surgery setting, laparoscopic exploration provides the opportunity to exclude or confirm a diagnosis as well as definitively manage the causative pathology without committing the patient to a laparotomy [1].

A.J. Tompeck
Trauma, Burn, and Surgical Critical Care Fellow, University of Texas Southwestern Medical Center, Department of Surgery, Dallas, TX, USA
e-mail: allison.tompeck@utsouthwestern.edu

M. Narayan (✉)
Acute Care Surgery/Surgical Intensive Care Unit/Department of Surgery, University of Texas Southwestern Medical Center, Department of Surgery, Dallas, TX, USA
e-mail: mayur.Narayan@gmail.com

Successful implementation of laparoscopic exploration mandates preoperative planning, standardization of personnel, operating room setup, and expedited mobilization of laparoscopic equipment. The purpose of this chapter is to outline the feasibility of laparoscopic exploration of free air, the steps involved, and associated indications and contraindications and finally discuss the risks and benefits of this procedure.

General Technique

Preparation

It is absolutely imperative that the surgeon understands and assesses the local environment and resources available to perform this procedure. Even quaternary hospitals with full expertise face challenges performing this procedure during off hours, particularly nights and weekends. The importance of operating room setup, patient positioning, and expedient access to laparoscopic instruments is paramount. Proper preparation of the operating room will facilitate a successful, safe, and timely surgery. Furthermore, standardization of a laparoscopic setup promotes efficiency and limits disturbances throughout the procedure [4]. It is also important to "fly ahead of the jet" and anticipate instruments potentially required for a given procedure, thereby limiting frustration and promoting productivity. For example, for a morbidly obese patient (BMI > 35), an extra long/bariatric instrument set should be in the room [4].

Key personnel include the anesthesiologist, surgeon, surgical technologist, and circulating nurse. It is imperative that each member be familiar with the operating room setup and steps of laparoscopic exploration. The anesthesia provider must maintain continuous communication with the surgeon regarding hemodynamic stability and cardiopulmonary status [5]. It is the surgeon's responsibility to ensure the anesthesiologist is aware of the potential pitfalls of laparoscopy

Fig. 2.1 Laparoscopic room setup (Reprinted with permission from *Zeni TM, Frantzides CT, Moore RE, 2009* (Zani TM, Frantzides CT, Moore RE (2009). Endosuite Configuration [Photograph]. Retrieved from https://www-clinicalkey-com.foyer.swmed.edu/#!/content/book/3-s2.0-B9781416041085500396))

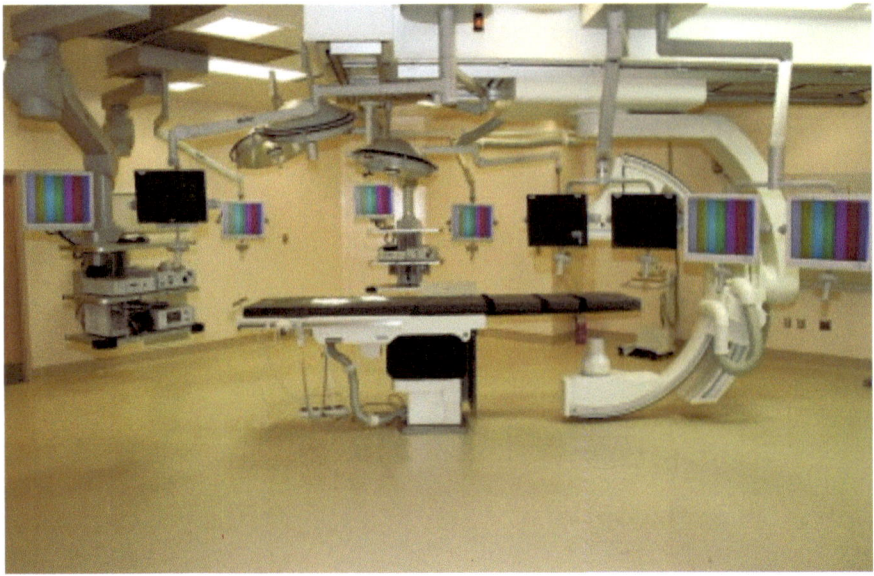

in the emergent setting. The surgical technologist is also a critical member of the team. A working knowledge of laparoscopic surgical instruments, staplers, energy devices (harmonic, ligasure etc.), and needle drivers is mandatory and will facilitate ease of operation. Finally, a circulating nurse must be able to quickly retrieve instruments and equipment as well as troubleshoot device and monitor malfunctions.

Operating Room Setup

The operating room should comfortably accommodate at least two monitors and laparoscopic equipment in a manner that permits unobstructed movement around the surgical field. Place the primary monitor directly across from the primary surgeon at eye level and a secondary monitor opposite the first assistant. As a rule, the surgeon, operative field, and monitor should align to optimize eye-hand coordination and economy of movement [2]. Position the insufflator, light source, cautery, and energy sources (e.g., Harmonic, etc.) in a single laparoscopic stack, which can rotate around the operating room table (Fig. 2.1).

Patient Positioning

Position the patient on the operating room table in the supine position. Following induction of general endotracheal anesthesia, secure the patient with two adjustable straps at the mid-thigh and mid-chest in anticipation of various intraoperative positions [4]. Alternatively, or for pelvic pathology, place a beanbag beneath the patient and a safety strap across

Table 2.1 Specific patient positions

Procedure	Position
Hiatal hernia	Supine, split leg
Perforated ulcers	Supine, split leg
Appendectomy	Supine
Hernia (inguinal, ventral)	Supine
Small and large bowel perforation	Supine
Pelvic (colorectal, gynecologic)	Supine, lithotomy

the chest to prevent the patient from slipping. This not only secures the patient but also provides flexibility for different table positions. The addition of a footboard is a useful adjunct if steep reverse Trendelenburg is anticipated or if the patient has a BMI > 35 [3]. Although not required for all cases, decompressing the stomach and bladder with nasogastric tube and Foley catheter accordingly is recommended. Finally, a patient's position is also dependent upon surgeon preference and underlying pathology. Table 2.1 lists common positions for a given laparoscopic surgical procedure.

In lithotomy position, the pelvis should rest at the break of the table for unobstructed access to the perineum and rectum. Place each leg in adjustable stirrups, and pad bony prominences, tubes, or cords. Abduct the legs to a 20–25° position with thighs slightly above or level to the abdomen. Tuck the patient's arm in the anatomic position thereby allowing the surgeon to move cephalad and maintain full range of motion (Fig. 2.2a). Again, be sure to use ample padding around potential pressure points and provide anesthesia access to intravenous lines or monitors [2]. Finally, consider ergonomics and the interface of the operative equipment, patient position, surgeon position, and laparoscopic instruments.

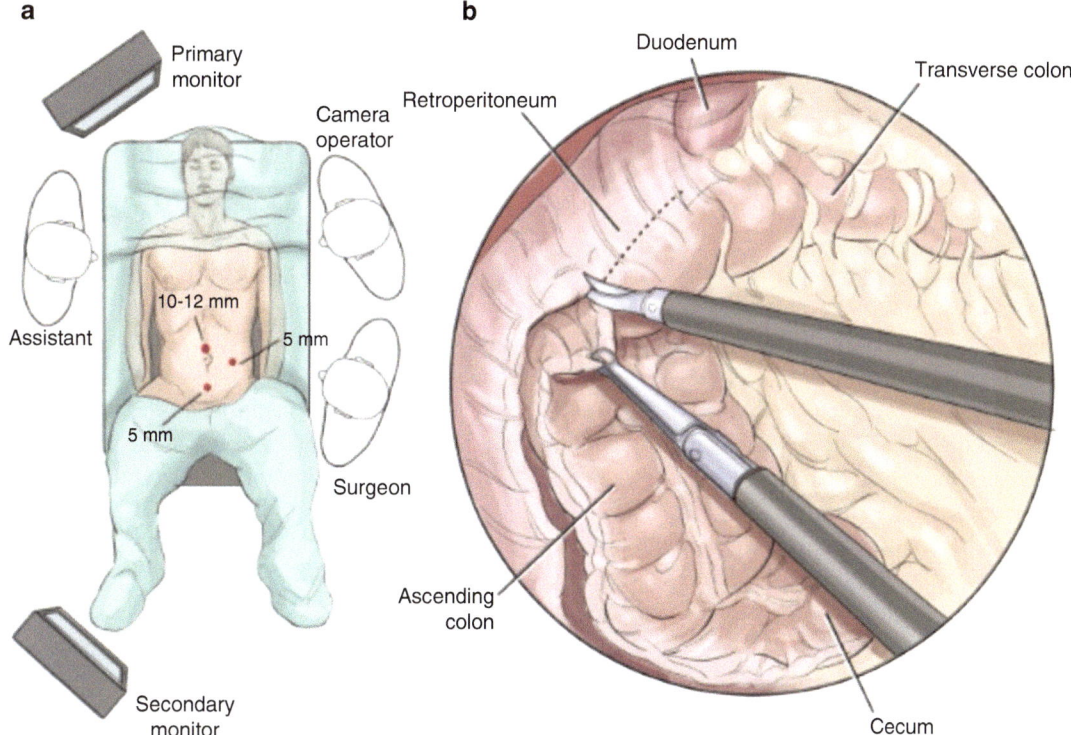

Fig. 2.2 (a) Lithotomy with arms tucked. (b) Hepatic flexure takedown (Reprinted with permission from *Cima RR, Pemberton JH, 2013*.(Cima RR, Pemberton JH (2013). Figure 59.6 [Image]. Retrieved from https://www-clinicalkey-com.foyer.swmed.edu/#!/content/book/3-s2.0-B9781416041092000593)

Equipment

A basic laparoscopic instrument set varies between institutions and is tailored to surgeon preference. However, at minimum, a laparoscopic set should include the following: 5 or 10 mm angled laparoscope (30° or 45°), graspers (including two nontraumatic bowel graspers), scissors, and a suction irrigator [2, 4]. Additional 5 and 10 mm trocars should be readily available. Consider each differential diagnosis and anticipate specific instruments potentially required.

Procedure

Access

Access into the abdominal cavity is achieved by one of three different techniques: insertion of Veress needle, direct blind trocar placement with an optical port, or open approach (Hasson) [6]. The Hasson technique with cutdown and direct visualization of primary trocar placement is associated with decreased risk of trocar-related complications, particularly in patients with prior abdominal surgery. The umbilicus is con-veniently attached to the underlying fascia, which assists in elevation of the fascia and peritoneum away from abdominal viscera [6]. However, if prior midline abdominal surgery precludes periumbilical entry, another site may be selected. Palmers point, located 3 cm below the costal margin in the midclavicular line, is a safe alternative for Veress needle placement to obtain insufflation [3, 6]. Following placement of a 5 mm (or 10 mm if using Hasson technique) trocar, the peritoneal cavity is insufflated with carbon dioxide to a pressure of 8–12 mm Hg and up to 15 mm Hg as tolerated.

Steps

A 5 mm or 10 mm angled laparoscope is inserted through the trocar to begin exploration and facilitate placement of secondary trocars. The surgeon must remember that the first step in any laparoscopic procedure is to insure no injury has occurred during abdominal entry.

The number and location of additional ports are based upon presumed intra-abdominal pathology and planned intervention. When placing additional trocars, utilize the angle of the laparoscope to visualize the undersurface of the abdominal wall and avoid the superior and inferior epigastric vessels running within the rectus sheath, immediately posterior to the rectus abdominis muscle. Surgeons are reminded that optimal trocar placement is one handbreath apart to avoid superseding of instruments. The principle of triangulation must be maintained to facilitate ease of abdominal exploration.

Exploring the Upper Abdomen

Place the table in steep reverse Trendelenburg, allowing gravity to assist with caudal retraction of the viscera, and begin in the epigastrium [4]. Retract the left lateral lobe of the liver in the anterior lateral direction. This can be done using a blunt atraumatic grasper. Survey the diaphragmatic hiatus, gastroesophageal junction, anterior stomach, and gastrohepatic ligament. The lesser sac can be accessed directly through the foramen of Winslow following dissection through the gastrohepatic ligament or by division of the gastrocolic and gastrosplenic ligaments. The latter is achieved by gently elevating the anterior stomach and greater omentum, while the transverse colon falls posteriorly. The gastrocolic ligament is divided by using an energy source in a direction parallel to the greater curvature, and visualization of the posterior stomach confirms entry into the correct space.

Next, rotate the bed toward the left to examine the contents of the right upper quadrant including the gastrocolic omentum, hepatic flexure, and gallbladder. Division of the hepatocolic ligament will release the hepatic flexure for improved exposure (Fig. 2.2b). To perform kocherization of the duodenum, free the lateral and posterior peritoneal attachments of the duodenum with a combination of sharp and blunt dissection. Sweep the duodenum medially to expose the posterior wall and pancreatic head.

Rotate the bed to the right, with the patients left side up and continue into the left upper quadrant. Transection of the splenocolic ligament provides mobilization of the colon and improved examination. Previous division of the gastrosplenic and gastrocolic ligaments expedites this step. It is important to remember that any omentum adherent to the spleen must be dissected sharply, as aggressive retraction will lead to splenic injury and intra-abdominal hemorrhage.

Exploration of the Lower Abdomen

Return the bed to the neutral position and elevate the greater omentum between two atraumatic graspers toward the anterior abdominal wall. This maneuver exposes the transverse colon and simultaneously partitions the abdomen. Gently place the greater omentum and transverse colon in the upper abdomen and maintain retraction in the cephalad direction. Transition the table into steep Trendelenburg with the left side up. Sweep the small intestine out of the pelvis to explore the sigmoid colon, rectum, bladder, and inguinal-femoral space. Of note, the descending and sigmoid colon is tethered by its blood supply. Apply gentle countertraction to straighten and expose the colon as well as the associated mesocolon. If needed, perform mobilization of lateral attachments of the colon along the line of Toldt.

While in steep Trendelenburg, rotate the bed in the opposite direction and sweep the small intestine toward the left hemiabdomen. Examine the cecum, distal ileum, ascending colon, bladder, and inguinal-femoral space. Tent up the ileocecal mesentery and mobilize the lateral attachments as needed.

Once completed, identify the ileocecal valve, and with two atraumatic graspers, examine the small bowel in 10 cm segments moving proximally toward the ligament of Treitz. As the middle third of the small bowel is approached, eliminate the Trendelenburg position and return the patient to a neutral position.

Upon completion of the procedure, secondary trocars are removed under direct visualization and each site observed for bleeding. Laparoscopic ports of 10 mm or greater should be closed to prevent trocar site hernias, with a suture on a curved needle or using a closure device such as the Gore-Tex Suture Passer, Carter-Thomason Device, or Endoclosure Suture Device. Regardless of the technique selected, the abdominal fascia should be clearly identified and closed in a tension-free manner.

Adjuncts

Methylene blue can be instilled via a nasogastric tube or Foley catheter to study the integrity of the foregut or bladder accordingly. Typically 1% methylene blue is diluted in normal saline to a volume adequate for distention of the stomach, duodenum, or bladder. Another helpful tool is intraoperative esophagogastroduodenoscopy (EGD) for investigation of stomach and small bowel pathology. Both methylene blue and EGD can also be used to evaluate a repair or anastomosis upon completion. Placement of a hand port provides the option of manual manipulation without full conversion to laparotomy [2]. These ports maintain insufflation while simultaneously allowing for retraction and dissection. In patients with free air secondary to mesenteric ischemia and perforation, newer technologies such as Pinpoint offer real-time fluorescent imaging of vasculature and intestinal structures.

Conversion: When and Why?

Conversion to open procedure should be pursued at the surgeon's discretion based upon intra-abdominal findings, unclear anatomy, or surgeon experience and comfort [2, 7].

Other commonly cited indications for conversion are the following: inability to establish pneumoperitoneum, lack of progress, uncontrolled intra-abdominal bleeding, cardiopulmonary instability, and instrument or equipment issues [7]. Inability to establish pneumoperitoneum is encountered in the presence of ascites, organomegaly, or late-stage pregnancy [2]. All of these scenarios are causes for concern and should prompt reevaluation of this approach. As discussed later in the chapter, preoperative hemodynamic lability is a contraindication to laparoscopic exploration given the potential negative effects of insufflation. In addition, induction of pneumoperitoneum and exaggerated patient positioning may worsen hemodynamic lability. Of note, at no point is conversion considered a failure of the case but rather a change in operative strategy.

Indications

For the purpose of this chapter, the main indication for laparoscopic exploration is pneumoperitoneum of unknown etiology. In this instance, clinical and radiographic information is indicative of free intraperitoneal air without identification of the specific underlying pathology [5]. However, clinical clues imbedded within the history, physical exam, and radiographs will narrow differential diagnoses and guide diagnostic laparoscopy. In addition, depending on the surgeon's experience and proficiency with advanced laparoscopy, definitive surgical management can be safely accomplished as well.

Current evidence demonstrates that laparoscopy is both safe and effective when employed in the acute care setting. Common causes of pneumoperitoneum successfully treated at the time of laparoscopic exploration are perforated diverticulitis, perforated peptic ulcer disease, small bowel perforation, and large bowel perforation [4, 5]. Other less common etiologies include perforated cholecystitis, perforated appendicitis, complicated Meckel's diverticulum, postoperative anastomotic failure, acute incarceration of paraesophageal hernia, and traumatic injury [1, 8].

Contraindications

The main contraindication to laparoscopic exploration is hemodynamic instability [9]. Insufflation elevates intra-abdominal pressure and compresses the collapsible inferior vena cava, which decreases venous return and cardiac output. Insufficient visceral perfusion ensues with a worsening metabolic lactic acidosis. In patients with underlying shock and instability, insufflation may prompt progression into irreversible cardiovascular collapse. Relative contraindica-

Table 2.2 Contraindications to laparoscopic exploration

Anesthesia
Inability to tolerate general anesthesia
Comorbidities (e.g., increased intracranial pressure)
Procedure
Extensive previous intra-abdominal surgeries ("frozen")
Inability to tolerate a laparotomy
Bleeding diathesis

tions are divided into two categories: anesthesia and procedure related (Table 2.2). The inability to tolerate general anesthesia will limit laparoscopy as an option for intra-abdominal evaluation. Certain comorbidities, such as increased intracranial pressure, decompensated congestive heart failure, or uncontrolled hypercapnic respiratory failure, are unlikely to tolerate insufflation [6]. Bleeding diathesis, commonly listed as a contraindication, may be overcome with the advent of various laparoscopic energy devices (e.g., Harmonic, Argon Beam, etc.) and topical hemostatic agents (e.g., Floseal, Everest, Nu-Knit, Surgicel, etc.) [1, 4].

Risks

The risk of delaying diagnosis or missing underling pathology during laparoscopy is of highest concern. It cannot be overemphasized that the decision to undertake laparoscopic evaluation should be driven by surgical expertise and confidence in thorough evaluation of the entire abdomen [5].

Injuries suffered upon entry into the abdomen are uncommon but nonetheless infer morbidity and mortality. Although the risk is dependent upon method of entry, major vascular and bowel injuries occur in between 0.04% and 0.18% of procedures [6]. Vascular injuries include abdominal wall hematomas, retroperitoneal hematomas, port site bleeding, and direct injury to a named vessel.

Risks can also be attributed to the physiologic consequence of inducing pneumoperitoneum as well as intraoperative positioning, particularly reverse Trendelenburg [6]. As mentioned in the previous chapter, the increase in intra-abdominal pressure reduces venous return, preload, and ultimately cardiac output [3, 6]. This is especially important in the setting of hypovolemia, which is potentially ameliorated with preoperative resuscitation. In addition, insufflation stretches the peritoneal lining causing vagal nerve stimulation and bradyarrhythmias [3, 6]. Treatment should begin with cessation of the procedure, urgent evacuation of the pneumoperitoneum, and returning the patient to a neutral position. ACLS protocol is then implemented as necessary.

From a respiratory standpoint, insufflation impedes diaphragmatic excursion, increases airway pressures, and decreases both FRC and compliance [3]. Hypoxemia can also result from intrapulmonary shunting and VQ mismatch [6]. An experienced anesthesiologist will counteract these issues by increasing the tidal volume and positive end expiratory pressure (PEEP).

Another catastrophic complication of laparoscopic surgery is CO_2 embolization to the right outflow tract resulting in cardiopulmonary collapse [6]. Treatment includes evacuation of pneumoperitoneum, placing patient in Trendelenburg position, aspiration of gas from the right internal jugular vein, and supportive measures. Traditionally, patients were transitioned to the left lateral position for evacuation of CO_2; however, recent guidelines have questioned the safety of this step.

Other risks associated with specific laparoscopic procedures will be addressed in the according chapter.

Benefits

General

Laparoscopic exploration for pneumoperitoneum provides the opportunity for thorough examination of the abdominal cavity and confirmation of a diagnosis in 85–100% of cases [8]. If laparoscopic exploration cannot be completed adequately or open intervention is required, three options remain: traditional laparotomy, minilaparotomy, and hand-assisted laparoscopy. The latter two are directed by intra-abdominal findings during laparoscopy and are associated with improved outcomes. In cases of occult or small volume pneumoperitoneum, laparoscopic exploration will minimize the rate of nontherapeutic laparotomies [5].

Immune System

Postoperative morbidity is frequently a manifestation of the immune stress response to surgery and its relationship to the patients underlying immune competence. Numerous articles have demonstrated preserved immune function and improved surgical stress response following laparoscopy as compared to open procedures [9]. This concept is well demonstrated in a randomized trial of colorectal patients, showing that human leukocyte antigen-DR function remains elevated following laparoscopic colorectal surgery and predicts expedited recovery [10]. In emergency general surgery and in patients with peritonitis, open surgery increases the incidence of bacteremia and systemic inflammation leading to transiently impaired immunologic defenses as compared to laparoscopic procedures [5, 9]. Conceptually, minimally invasive surgery has the

potential to minimize tissue trauma, which ultimately endorses a robust and efficient immune response and recovery [2].

Patient Populations

Incisional pain is of particular importance in the elderly population and associated with both pulmonary and cardiovascular consequences [9]. Low tidal volume respiration can lead to atelectasis and in worse cases pneumonia, which increases postoperative morbidity and mortality. Pain also limits patient mobility and thereby increases the risk of venous thromboembolism. As an example, transhiatal or transthoracic hiatal hernia repair in elderly is associated with significant morbidity and mortality. However, if the same repair can be accomplished laparoscopically, either electively or emergently, evidence shows improve outcomes and decreased postoperative pain.

Conclusion

Laparoscopic exploration of free air is a safe and feasible operative technique. The success of this procedure is dependent upon awareness, standardization, and experience. Surgeon's expertise and comfort with advanced laparoscopy is the primary variable for a successful outcome. Operating room setup, laparoscopic trays, and team familiarity with the procedure provides the foundation for each operation. Every step of the operation from patient positioning to induction of anesthesia to port placement must be both thoughtful and decisive. Patient safety is of utmost importance and is facilitated through clear concise communication between the anesthesiologist and surgeon. Again, conversion to open does not represent failure but a change in strategy. The principles and standards of acute care surgery prevail, regardless of the approach or indication. However, laparoscopic exploration for free air provides the opportunity for diagnosis and intervention through minimally invasive techniques associated with decreased postoperative complications, decreased morbidity, and immune competence.

With the advent of laparoscopic courses including Fundamentals of Laparoscopic Surgery (FLS), Fundamentals of Endoscopic Surgery (FES), and Fundamental Use of Surgical Energy (FUSE) and support of organizations such as American College of Surgeons (ACS) and Society of American Gastrointestinal and Endoscopic Surgeons (SAGES), surgeons will become increasingly more comfortable with a laparoscopic approach to free air. Furthermore, experience among surgeons will eventually shift the paradigm from simple diagnosis to advanced therapeutic management.

Take-Home Messages

1. Successful laparoscopic exploration starts with pre-operative planning, standardization of personnel, and operative room setup.
2. Open communication between anesthesia and surgical teams regarding the hemodynamic effects of pneumoperitoneum promotes patient safety and will guide surgical decision-making throughout the procedure.
3. Laparoscopic exploration includes abdominal entry, examination of peritoneal surfaces, intra-abdominal organ, and free peritonea fluid with the use of adjuncts as indicated.
4. Laparoscopic exploration for free air is safe and feasible.

References

1. Memon MA, Fitzgibbons RJ. The role of minimal access surgery in the acute abdomen. Surg Clin N Am. 1997;77:1333–53.
2. Bittner JG, Rabl C, Campos GM. Technical aspects of laparoscopic surgery. In: Ashley SW, editor. Scientific American Surgery. 2015. Retrieved from https://www.deckerip.com/decker/scientific-american-surgery/chapter/481/.
3. Gould JC, Simon K. Principles and techniques of abdominal access and physiology of pneumoperitoneum. In: Ashley SW, editor. Scientific American Surgery. 2015. Retrieved from https://www.deckerip.com/decker/scientific-american-surgery/chapter/480/
4. Tsuda ST. Introduction to laparoscopic operations. In: Fischer JE, editor. Fischer's mastery of surgery. Philadelphia: Lippincott Williams & Wilkins; 2012. p. 847–53.
5. Navez B, Navez J. Laparoscopy in the acute abdomen. Best Pract Res Clin Gastroenterol. 2014;28:3–17.
6. Graham JA, Jackson PG. Laparoscopic Surgery. In: Evans SRT, editor. Surgical Pitfalls: Prevention and Management (Chapter 7). 2009. Retrieved from http://www.surgicalcore.org/chapter/85642.
7. Agresta F, Campanile FC, Podda M, et al. Current status of laparoscopy for acute abdomen in Italy:a critical appraisal of 2012 clinical guidelines from two consecutive nationwide surveys with analysis of 271, 323 cases over 5 years. Surg Endosc. 2017;31(4):1785–95. doi: 10.1007/s00464-016-5175-4. Epub 2016 Aug 29.
8. Sauerland S, Agresta F, Bergamaschi R, et al. Laparoscopy for abdominal emergencies: evidenced-based guidelines of the European Association for Endoscopic Surgery. Surg Endosc. 2006;20:14–29.
9. Saverio SD. Emergency laparoscopy: a new emerging discipline for treating abdominal emergencies attempting to minimize costs and invasiveness and maximize outcomes and patients' comfort. J Trauma Acute Care Surg. 2014;77:338–50.
10. Veenhof AAFA, Vlug MS, van der Pas MHGM, et al. Surgical stress response and postoperative immune function after laparoscopy or open surgery with fast track or standard perioperative care. Ann Surg. 2012;255:216–21.

Suggested Readings

1. Sanabria A, Villegas MI, Morales Uribe CH. Laparoscopic repair for perforated peptic ulcer disease (review). Cochrane Database Syst Rev. 2013;2
2. Matsevych OY, Koto MZ, Motilall SR, et al. The role of laparoscopy in management of stable patients with penetrating abdominal trauma and organ evisceration. J Trauma Acute Care Surg. 2016;81:307–11.
3. Gagne DJ, Malay MB, Hogl NJ, Fowler DL. Bedside diagnostic Minilaparoscopy in the intensive care patient. Surgery. 2002;131(5):491–6.
4. Pecoraro AP, Cacchione RN, Sayad P, William ME, Ferzli GS. The routine use of diagnostic laparoscopy in the intensive care unit. Surg Endosc. 2001;15(7):638–41.
5. Kelly JJ, Puyana JC, Callery MP, Yood SM, Sandor A, Litwin DE. The feasibility and accuracy of diagnostic laparoscopy in the septic ICU patient. Surg Endosc. 2000;14(7):617–21.
6. Orlando R, Crowell KL. Laparoscopy in the critically ill. Surg Endosc. 1997;11(11):1072–4.
7. Walsh RM, Popovich MJ, Hoadley J. Bedside diagnostic laparoscopy and peritoneal lavage in the intensive care unit. Surg Endosc. 1998;12(12):1405–9.
8. Brandt CP, Priebe PP, Eckhauser ML. Diagnostic laparoscopy in the intensive care patient. Avoiding the nontherapeutic laparotomy. Surg Endosc. 1993;7(3):168–72.
9. Brandt CP, Priebe PP, Jacobs DG. Value of laparoscopy in trauma ICU patients with suspected acute acalculous cholecystitis. Surg Endosc. 1994;8(5):361–4. discussion 364–5.
10. Jaramillo EJ, Trevino JM, Berghoff KR, Franklin ME Jr. Bedside diagnostic laparoscopy in the intensive care unit: a 13-year experience. JSLS. 2006;10(2):155–9.
11. Hackert T, Kienle P, Weitz J, Werner J, Szabo G, Hagl S, Büchler MW, Schmidt J. Accuracy of diagnostic laparoscopy for early diagnosis of abdominal complications after cardiac surgery. Surg Endosc. 2003;17(10):1671–4.
12. Almeida J, Sleeman D, Sosa JL, Puente I, McKenney M, Martin L. Acalculous cholecystitis: the use of diagnostic laparoscopy. J Laparoendosc Surg. 1995;5(4):227–31.
13. Guidelines for Diagnostic Laparoscopy. https://www.sages.org/publications/guidelines/guidelines-for-diagnostic-laparoscopy/. Published 2002. Updated April 2012. Accessed February 19, 2017.

Ciara R. Huntington and B. Todd Heniford

Introduction

Incidence

Abdominal wall hernias are one of the most frequently encountered surgical diagnoses for acute care surgeons, with surgeons in the United States performing more than 360,000 ventral hernia repairs and 770,000 inguinal hernia repairs annually [1]. Inguinal hernias represent the majority of abdominal wall hernias; as many as one in four men and one in 50 women will require an inguinal hernia repair in their lifetime [2, 3]. The incidence of emergent hernia repairs, however, is increasing with a rise from 16.0 repairs per 100,000 person-years in 2001 to 19.2 per 100,000 person-years in 2010, with the majority of these occurring in patients 65 years and older [2]. Women have higher rates of incarcerated femoral hernias, while men have higher rates of emergent inguinal hernia repairs [2, 3]. As the population ages, incisional hernia repairs are also becoming more frequent, with an annual incidence of 23.5 per 100,000 person-years for women and 32.5 per 100,000 person-years for men [2].

Risk Factors and Pathophysiology: Inguinal and Ventral Hernias

Inguinal hernias have a bimodal peak, with indirect hernias more common in the pediatric age group (peak age 0–5) and direct in elderly adults (peak age 75–80). Indirect hernias are congenital, resulting from a patent processus vaginalis, which allows herniation of abdominal contents through the inguinal canal, and are more common in men than women [4]. Direct hernias appear in Hesselbach's triangle (bounded by the rectus abdominis/median arcuate ligament, inferior epigastric vessels, and inguinal ligament) secondary to a weakening in the abdominal wall [4]. Key risk factors for hernia formation include older age, abdominal obesity, genetics, repetitive straining of the abdominal muscles as with heavy lifting or coughing, collagen deficiencies, and nutritional status.

Ventral hernias are most commonly "incisional" hernias, occurring after a previous operation has weakened the patient's fascia. Incisional hernias may occur in the setting of wound infection, obesity, poor glucose control, tobacco use, malnutrition, and suboptimal surgical technique, and can affect up to 30% of laparotomies [5–7]. Trocar site hernias are small-necked hernias that occur following laparoscopy. Due to the tight incarceration of bowel and abdominal contents through these small defects (usually 5 mm or 10 mm), repair is often undertaken. Umbilical hernias are a common type of primary ventral hernias, commonly found in both men and women, and developed from a failure of the closure of the umbilical defect found in infancy. Conditions such as ascites, pregnancy, and abdominal obesity can expand this fascial defect and lead to an umbilical hernia.

When to Repair

Untreated, all hernias tend to expand over time. Watchful waiting for asymptomatic inguinal hernia has been repeatedly demonstrated to be cost-effective and safe [8]. However, when inguinal hernias become symptomatic, repair is suggested [9]. However, patients who have their hernias repaired while asymptomatic or minimally symptomatic are less likely to have chronic discomfort [10]; this is true for both

C.R. Huntington
General Surgery Chief Resident, Carolinas Medical Center, Department of Surgery, Charlotte, NC, USA
e-mail: Ciara.huntington@carolinas.org

B.T. Heniford (✉)
Chief, Division of Gastrointestinal and Minimally Invasive Surgery, Carolinas Medical Center, Department of Surgery, Charlotte, NC, USA
e-mail: todd.heniford@carolinas.org

© Springer International Publishing AG 2018
K.A. Khwaja, J.J. Diaz (eds.), *Minimally Invasive Acute Care Surgery*, https://doi.org/10.1007/978-3-319-64723-4_3

inguinal and ventral hernias [11]. Given that inguinal hernias are a chronic problem, get bigger with time, and carry a small but real risk of incarceration, having a patient choose "a good time in their life" to repair the hernia electively is often appropriate. Due to the higher risk for incarceration, surgical repair of femoral hernias is indicated, even if asymptomatic [12].

Incarcerated hernias provide a more challenging picture for the surgeon, though minimally invasive approach can be safe and feasible in the correctly selected patients, even in the setting of strangulation [13–15].

Preoperative Diagnostic Workup

Inguinal and abdominal wall hernias are primarily diagnosed with careful history and physical exam. A careful examination should be undertaken with the patient standing and, possibly, supine. In examination of a groin hernia, the contralateral side should always be examined. In addition, a testicular examination in men and palpation for an asymptomatic umbilical defect should be a routine part of preoperative examination for groin hernias. A history of obstructive symptoms such as constipation should be elicited, in addition to questions about difficulty voiding and chronic cough.

Blood Work and Laboratory Workup

For healthy patients undergoing elective hernia repair, no routine bloodwork may be necessary. However, in the acute setting, for a patient who presents with incarcerated abdominal wall hernia, labs that may be appropriate include a basic metabolic panel to evaluate for electrolyte abnormalities and acute kidney injury, complete blood count to evaluate for leukocytosis and anemia, and a lactic acid level test. For patients whose hernias do not require immediate intervention, a hemoglobin A1c level can provide a useful baseline for blood glucose control prior to elective surgical repair [7].

Imaging

In the setting of an acute abdomen, an upright and supine abdominal x-ray series can demonstrate the presence of small bowel obstruction and pneumoperitoneum. For patients presenting with an acute incarceration of a groin hernia that is confirmed with physical exam, imaging is not required prior to proceeding to the operating room. When available, ultrasound may be helpful to discern possible incarcerated bowel versus incarcerated preperitoneal or omental fat. In small abdominal wall hernias such as trocar site hernias or umbilical hernias, physical exam may provide enough infor-

mation for the surgeon to forgo advancing imaging. However, for more complex abdominal wall hernias, CT scanning is useful in determining the presence of incarcerated bowel, number, location, and width of fascial defect(s) and helps to predict the need for advanced techniques such as component separation for fascial closure. In obese patients who present with pain and possibly incarcerated ventral incisional hernias, physical exam and ultrasound may not provide enough information, and CT scanning may offer more reliable information prior to surgical decision making. Finally, in those patients who present with small bowel obstruction from ventral hernia, close examination of the bowel and passage of oral contrast through incarcerated loops can help with planning for operative versus nonoperative management [16].

Management

Inguinal Hernia

In patients who present with a minimally symptomatic hernia that is reducible, watchful waiting may be appropriate. However, a patient with an incarcerated hernia may require prompt surgical attention depending on the clinical scenario. Patients may endorse acute, intractable groin pain; symptoms of small bowel obstruction such as nausea, vomiting, obstipation, and constipation; and an erythematous, irreducible groin bulge. If a hernia is freely reducible or an incarcerated hernia does not have the clinical signs of obstruction or strangulation, an elective repair may be scheduled, though patients with incarceration symptoms should be encouraged to undergo surgery.

If there is any concern for impending compromise of the bowel due to hernia incarceration, the patient should be taken to the operating room. Even if the hernia is successfully reduced, it is strongly recommended to visualize the incarcerated loop of bowel in the operating room, to ensure it is viable. If a patient presents with an acutely incarcerated hernia but has no evidence of strangulation, the bowel may be evaluated for viability according to the clinical scenario. Relieving the acute incarceration may provide time for rehydration and preoperative discussion and planning.

General exclusion criteria for a laparoscopic approach are shown in Table 3.1, but each patient's situation must be addressed individually. For patients with significant cardiopulmonary risk factors, inguinal hernia repair under local anesthesia is feasible in the emergent setting [17] but requires an open operative approach. Femoral hernias may be approached in a similar laparoscopic manner to inguinal hernias, recognized by a lump below the inguinal ligament.

The transabdominal preperitoneal (TAPP) inguinal hernia repair is the preferred laparoscopic approach as it allows for visualization and manipulation of the intraabdominal con-

Table 3.1 General exclusion and conversion criteria – laparoscopic hernia repairs

Exclusion criteria – laparoscopic hernia repair
Insufficient surgeon experience with laparoscopic approach
Patient inability to tolerate general anesthesia
Recurrent hernias previously repaired laparoscopically may benefit from open approach
Fascial defects >10 cm
Criteria for conversation from laparoscopic to open
Hostile abdomen with inability to perform laparoscopic adhesiolysis
Inability to reduce incarcerated hernia contents despite described techniques
Loss of domain in the abdominal wall or patients with massive fascial defects where laparoscopic repair with intraperitoneal mesh is not feasible

tents in the incarcerated hernia. The use of the totally extraperitoneal (TEP) approach in emergent incarcerated hernia repair has been reported [19] but requires considerable surgeon experience in this approach. The disadvantage of such an approach is the lack of being able to directly reduce the entrapped hernia contents directly into the abdomen.

Operative Approach for Incarcerated Inguinal Hernias (TAPP)

Steps:

1. In the preoperative holding area, patients are often given 250 mg acetazolamide to assist with postoperative discomfort from carbon dioxide insufflation. Foley catheters, usually avoided in elective repairs, may be recommended for patients with incarcerated hernias. Preoperative cefazolin is provided within 1 hour (h) of incision.
2. The patient is taken to the operating room and placed in the supine position, and general endotracheal anesthesia is established. The entire abdomen, groin, and thigh are sterilely prepped and draped.
3. We choose to make an infraumbilical incision, and an open umbilical cutdown is performed to enter the abdomen with a laparoscopic cannula placed with the sharp inner cannula. If an umbilical hernia is encountered, a curvilinear incision is made around the hernia anteriorly and it is dissected circumferentially. Once the hernia is freed from the subcutaneous tissues, the hernia sac may be entered and contents reduced. A port can be placed through the hernia, if present, and then repaired at time of closure in the standard open fashion.
4. Two additional left and right 5 mm ports are placed under direct visualization lateral to the umbilical port, slightly above the umbilicus (Fig. 3.1). The umbilical port is upsized to a 10 mm port and a 10 mm camera is utilized.

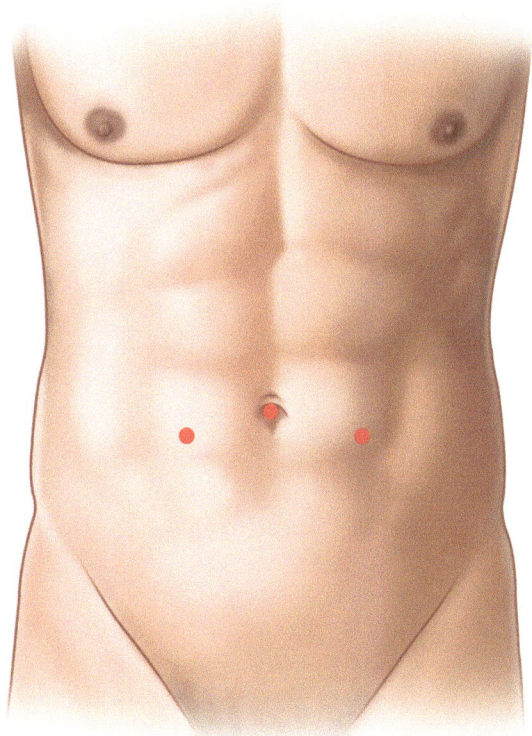

Fig. 3.1 Port placement for laparoscopic inguinal hernia repair. Two 5 mm trocars and a single 10 mm trocar, to accommodate a rolled mesh, are placed

5. Inspection of the abdomen is conducted. The site of the hernia and the contralateral side are closely inspected. The incarcerated contents are reduced into the peritoneal cavity with gentle laparoscopic retraction and pressure from the outside. The omentum and intestine are closely inspected following reduction.
6. The repair portion of the operation is started by cutting the peritoneum with a laparoscopic scissor at the medial umbilical ligament and proceeding laterally. Care should be taken not to start the incision too caudally. Another common mistake is extending the incision inferiorly, instead of laterally. The epigastric vessels must be visualized and avoided.
7. With a laparoscopic grasper, the peritoneal edge is grasped and retracted. Carefully, the peritoneum is swept down. Small vessels may be taken with sharp dissection with cautery, and all potential bleeding is carefully cauterized to preserve good visualization of dissection planes. A large peritoneal flap is created.
8. The dissection continued down to the pubis.
9. At this point, both a direct and indirect hernia can be visualized easily. With firm but gentle pressure, incarcerated hernia sac is reduced. "Walking" down the sac hand over

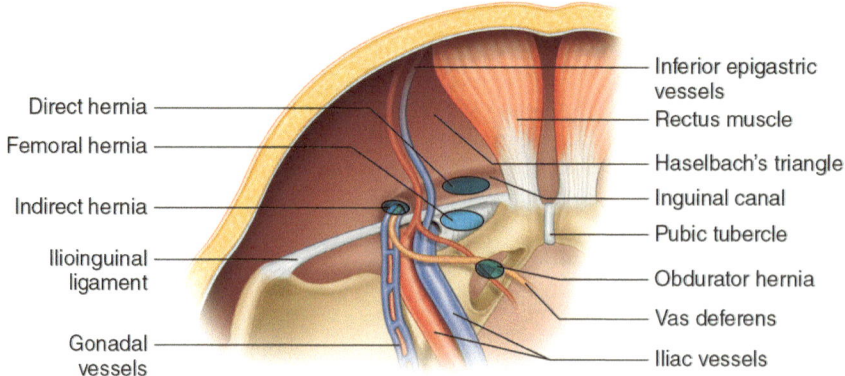

Fig. 3.2 Groin hernia anatomy and hernia types. Incarcerated direct, indirect, femoral, and obdurator hernias may all be approached from a laparoscopic approach with a thorough understanding of the anatomy

Direct hernia

Femoral hernia

Indirect hernia

Ilioinguinal ligament

Gonadal vessels

Inferior epigastric vessels

Rectus muscle

Haselbach's triangle

Inguinal canal

Pubic tubercle

Obdurator hernia

Vas deferens

Iliac vessels

hand with laparoscopic graspers will help apply tension as the attachments are peeled from the hernia sac.

Note: The femoral and obdurator spaces should also be identified and examined for incarcerated fat or herniated contents (Fig. 3.2).

10. For more difficult reductions, the patient may be placed in Trendelenburg position, and external pressure to reduce the hernia contents from the scrotum or inguinal canal can be applied as needed by an assistance. With meticulous technique, the fascia can be incised with laparoscopic scissors or hook cautery to facilitate reduction. Sharp dissection of the inguinal ring can be undertaken, with careful attention to surrounding vascular structures.

Note: As mentioned, after reduction, incarcerated bowel is carefully inspected for viability. Questionable viability should be observed for several minutes, as it can go from dusky to healthy as circulation is restored. If there is concern for bowel ischemia, the segment of bowel can be resected in a laparoscopic-assisted manner. The bowel is extracted via the umbilical trocar site with a wound protector in place. Standard bowel resection and anastomosis are performed, and the bowel is then returned to the abdomen. In situations like this, the peritoneum can be closed laparoscopically, and the inguinal hernia repair can be then performed via an open inguinal incision in order to place mesh outside of the potentially contaminated abdominal cavity. The advantages of this approach are avoiding a midline laparotomy altogether and also avoiding extracting potentially contaminated bowel via the inguinal incision. In the setting of contamination, primary suture repair of the fascial defect via an open or, perhaps, a laparoscopic approach is possible. In order to perform a primary suture repair via laparoscopy, a figure-of-eight stitch is placed to approximate shelving edge of the inguinal

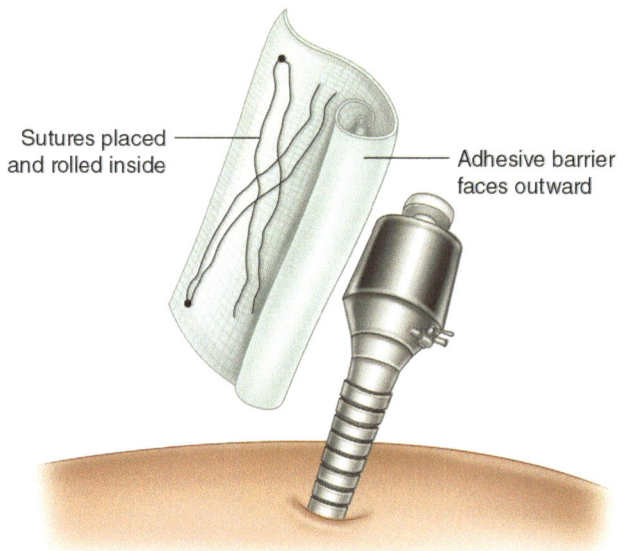

Sutures placed and rolled inside

Adhesive barrier faces outward

Fig. 3.3 Rolling mesh for introduction into the abdomen. When placing mesh inside the trocar, ensure the adhesive barrier faces outward, and sutures are rolled inside the mesh

ligament to the transversalis fascia, similar to an open McVay repair. Utilizing an extracorporeal knot tying in this instance can help tension the suture. The use of a biologic mesh may also be appropriate.

11. Preservation of the cord structures is attempted throughout the operation. Investigation of the cord structures for a cord lipoma is routinely conducted, and if presented, the lipoma is removed with careful dissection.
12. Generally, a large or extra-large contoured mesh is selected. The mesh is rolled and placed into the abdomen via the 10 mm trocar (Fig. 3.3).
13. The mesh is carefully laid in the preperitoneal space and laid flat against the abdominal wall. It is fixed to the

pubis with two or three tacks. We often placed a tack out laterally above the iliopubic tract (where the surgeon can palpate through the tip of the tacking device) and one in the rectus anteriorly. Tacks are not to be placed in the *triangle of doom* (an anatomical triangle defined by the vas deferens medially, spermatic vessels laterally, and external iliac vessels inferiorly) or the *triangle of pain* (an inverted "V"-shaped area with its apex at the internal inguinal ring and bounded by the iliopubic track anteriorly and by the testicular vessels posteromedially) (Fig. 3.2).

14. The peritoneum is closed with an absorbable suture in a running fashion or tacks.

Note: If a small hole is noted in the peritoneum, it is closed with an Endoloop or additional suture.

15. The ports are removed under direct vision to ensure there was no bleeding. The 10 mm trocar site fascia is closed with interrupted figure-of-eight 0 nonabsorbable sutures when a hernia is present and a #0 absorbable suture on an UR6 needle if not. When a hernia is present, the umbilical skin is tacked back down to the fascia with a 3–0 Monocryl.

16. The skin is closed with 4–0 Monocryl and Dermabond after injecting bupivacaine at each site, an ilioinguinal nerve block (Fig. 3.4) is also performed.

Incarcerated Ventral Hernias In patients who present with a mildly symptomatic incarcerated ventral hernia, watchful waiting may be appropriate. A repair can be conducted electively after preoperative risk stratification, and risk reduction

(weight loss, smoking cessation, blood glucose control) has been conducted. However, prompt surgery must be strongly encouraged in patients who endorse acute, intractable pain with symptoms of small bowel obstruction such as nausea, vomiting, obstipation, and constipation or have an erythematous, irreducible bulge noted on exam. If a hernia is freely reducible or an incarcerated hernia does not have the clinical signs of obstruction or strangulation, an elective repair may be scheduled. If there is significant concern for impending compromise of the bowel due to hernia incarceration, the patient should be taken to the operating room. Table 3.1 gives guidance on exclusion/inclusion criteria for laparoscopy, but each patient's clinical scenario must be taken in context of their operative risk factors, hemodynamic status, and the surgeon's confidence in his or her laparoscopic ability. Ventral hernias in patients with fascial defects greater than 10 cm may be better suited to open repair [18].

Operative Approach
Steps:

1. In the preoperative holding area, patients are provided with preoperative cefazolin within 1 h of incision. If there is a high likelihood of conversation to an open procedure, an epidural catheter placement for pain control is discussed. Injection of the transversus abdominis space bilaterally with long-acting local anesthesia to conduct regional nerve blocks is another option for nonnarcotic pain relief.

2. After consent is confirmed, the patient is transported to the operating room and placed supine on the table. Sequential leg compression devices and a Foley catheter are placed. The abdomen is clipped, prepped, and draped in a sterile fashion. An alcohol scrub with 4 × 4 gauze is

Fig. 3.4 Ilioinguinal nerve block. Injection is made at the entrance of the ilioinguinal nerve into the inguinal canal near at the deep ring and then along the iliopubic tract

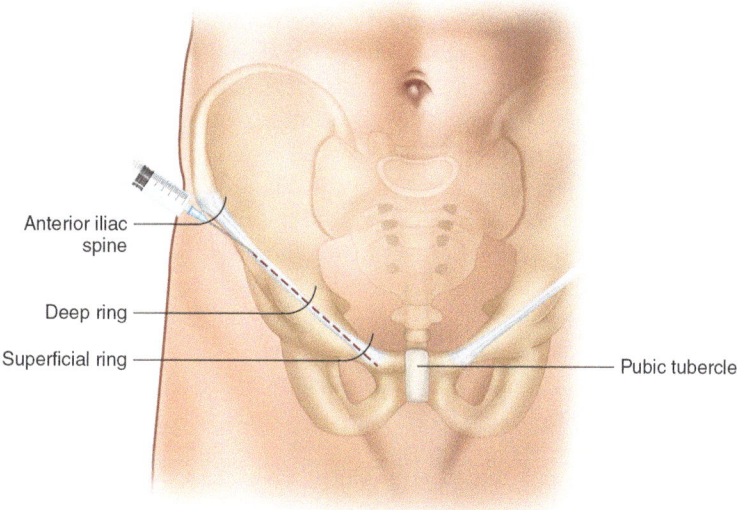

Anterior iliac spine

Deep ring

Superficial ring

Pubic tubercle

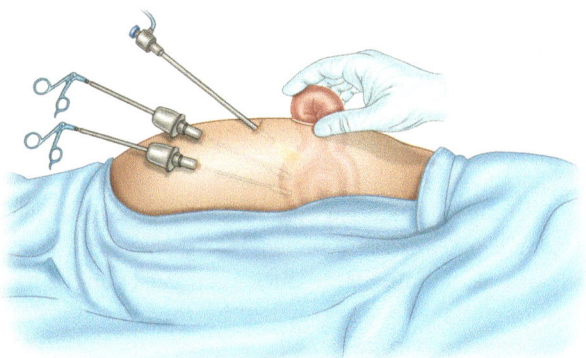

Fig. 3.6 Operative reduction of difficult incarcerated abdominal wall hernia. For a difficult laparoscopic hernia reduction, the surgeon may directly incise the skin over the hernia and perform a limited open dissection of the hernia sac with reduction of its contents. The hernia is then repaired in a laparoscopic-assisted open fashion with mesh

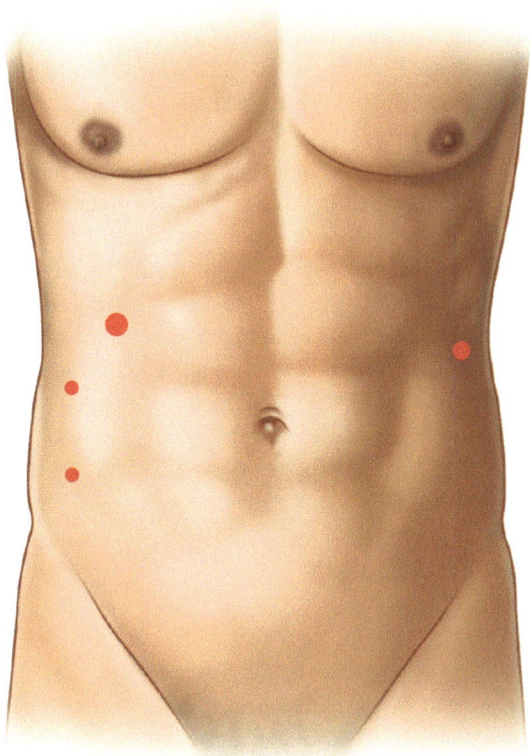

Fig. 3.5 Ventral hernia port placement. Laparoscopic port placement is important for successful ventral hernia repair. Additional 5 mm lateral ports can be added as necessary

routinely used to remove debris from the skin and assure hygiene prior to a chlorohexidine prep.

3. Using a 5 mm optical trocar, the peritoneum is entered in the location most appropriate for the patient's surgical history. Typically, a site in the right or left upper quadrant just off the costal margin is safely cannulated, and the abdomen is insufflated. Otherwise, a true cutdown through each layer of the abdominal wall can be performed.

4. Typically, two additional, 5 mm ports are placed on the lateral side of the abdomen under direct vision. An additional 5 mm port is often placed on the contralateral side (Fig. 3.5). One port is upsized to a 12 mm part to allow entry of the mesh. Site of laparoscopic port placement is important and depends on the hernia defect to be repaired and angles needed to take down adhesions and to allow tack placement into mesh on all sides. If a large ventral hernia is approached, additional lateral ports may be needed.

5. Another option for difficult laparoscopic hernia reduction and repair is to directly incise the skin over the hernia and perform a limited open dissection of the hernia sac with reduction of its contents (Fig. 3.6). A laparoscopic port can then be inserted under direct vision laterally, the hernia is closed, and additional ports are placed to fix the mesh (Fig. 3.7).

6. When performed truly laparoscopically, the adhesions are taken down sharply and meticulously with laparoscopic scissors to avoid injuries.

7. The incarcerated hernia is identified and reduced by steady, firm, though gentle, pressure. The hernia contents and sac are reduced by gentle downward laparoscopic traction, walking hand over hand with laparoscopic graspers, and manual pressure applied externally by an assistant.

8. If bowel is reduced, that is, worrisome for ischemia, it is observed for several minutes and if needed can be resected via an extraction site protected with a wound protector. However, a bowel resection for strangulation precludes the placement of synthetic mesh in most situations. Therefore, consideration of a laparoscopically placed biologic mesh or primary repair (without or without biologic mesh reinforcement) is undertaken.

Note: Primary repair can be undertaken via either open or laparoscopic approach. The laparoscopic approach is done via transfascial sutures passed with laparoscopic suture passer or by intracorporeal suturing of the defect. Intraabdominal insufflation pressure should be reduced when tensioning these sutures.

9. With the hernia reduced, the fascial defect is measured with spinal needles (placed through the skin/subcutaneous tissue to the edge of the fascial defect visualized laparoscopically) and an intraoperative silk suture as demonstrated in Fig. 3.8. This helps estimate the actual size of mesh needed regardless of the curvature of the patient's abdominal wall.

10. In the absence of contamination, a coated, synthetic mesh is selected, which should impede adhesions from the intestine. The center of the mesh is marked side to

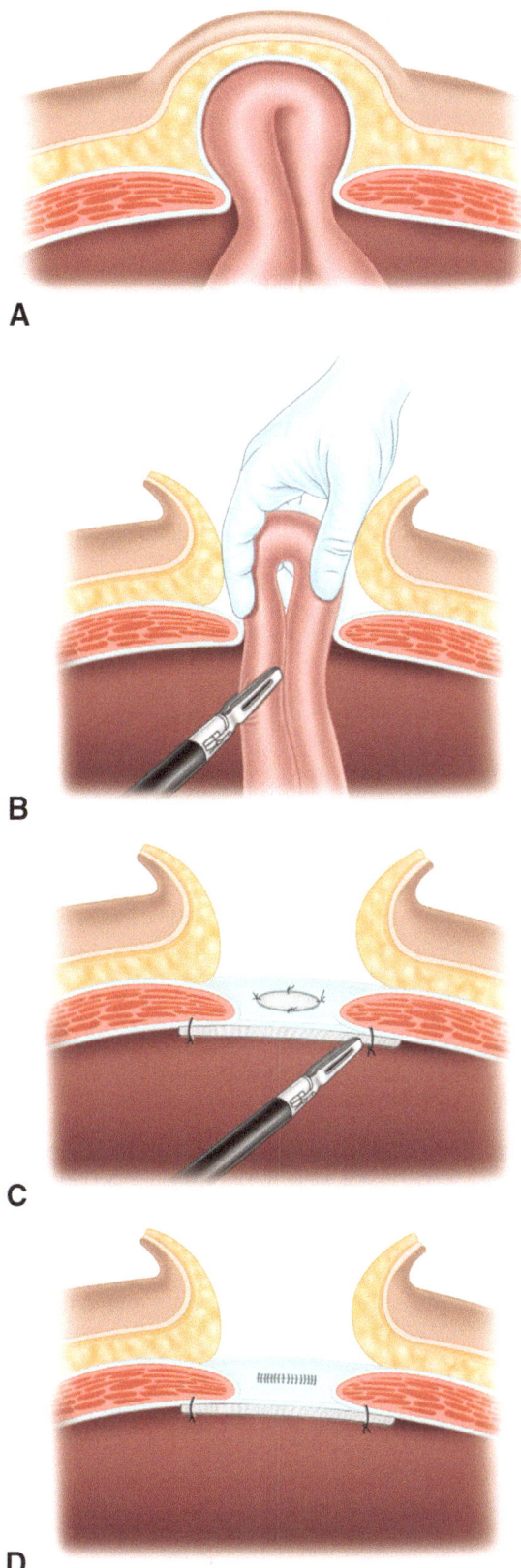

A

B

C

D

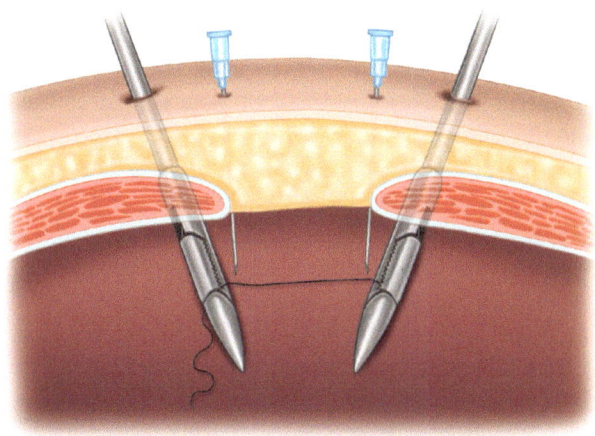

Fig. 3.8 Measuring the ventral hernia defect size intracorporeally. The fascial defect is measured with an intraoperative silk suture between spinal needles, placed through the skin/subcutaneous tissue to the edge of the fascial defect visualized laparoscopically. This estimates the actual size of mesh needed, regardless of the curvature of the patient's abdominal wall

side and head to foot with marking pens to aid with intraoperative positioning. The mesh is rolled and inserted through the 12 mm port. The mesh is then elevated using soft bowel graspers and positioned with the center of the mesh directly at the center of the fascial defect. The four quadrants of the mesh are secured using a tacker. Once these four points were secured, the remainder of the mesh is tacked circumferentially.

11. Typically, between four and eight permanent size-0 transfascial sutures are used to additionally secure the mesh around the fascial defect itself with assistance of a laparoscopic suture passer. Gor-Tex sutures may be substituted if desired. These are tied down and cut below the skin level, with the subcutaneous tissues "popped" up with a hemostat to avoid unsightly indentation. The mesh should be tight and well secured circumferentially.

12. The 12 mm balloon port site is closed using a 0 absorbable on a suture passer in figure-of-eight fashion.

13. The abdomen is desufflated and ports removed under direct visualization. The skin is closed using subcuticular 4–0 Monocryl at all port sites.

Postoperative Care

Patients with incarcerated, emergent hernia repairs are at increased risk for morbidity and mortality [13, 18, 20, 21], though the risk of mesh-related complications is equivalent if bowel resection is not required [16]. Postoperatively, all hernia patients are monitored for signs of infection or missed bowel injury. Patients with an acutely incarcerated hernia in the setting of advanced age, lactic acidosis, tenuous cardiopulmonary status, or extensive comorbidities are admitted to the intensive

Fig. 3.7 Laparoscopic-assisted reduction and repair of incarcerated ventral hernia. (**a**) Incarcerated ventral hernia with a small fascial defect. (**b**) Laparoscopic-assisted open reduction of the hernia. Patient may be placed in Trendelenburg and external pressure applied to reduce the hernia. (**c**) Laparoscopic-assisted placement of coated mesh with excellent mesh-to-defect ratio allows for a durable repair of hernia. (**d**) Open closure of fascial defect

care unit. Multimodal pain therapy is encouraged, with use of nonsteroidal agents, acetaminophen, and neuropathic pain medications in addition to oral narcotics. We do not routinely use nasogastric tubes, even in patients who have undergone bowel resections; however, NG tubes may be placed to treat severe postoperative ileus as needed. Seromas are universal after laparoscopic ventral repair, and patients should be counseled accordingly; we do not routinely leave drains in place. Wound complications, postoperative ileus, pneumonia, and acute kidney injury are the most common postoperative complications noted [14, 17]. A laparoscopic approach, however, appears to minimize the risk of wound complications, especially for obese and diabetic patients [22]. In patients with incarcerated bowel or after resection, patients should demonstrate some return of bowel function prior to discharge home. Follow-up is conducted 2–4 weeks after surgery. Patients should not lift greater than 20 pounds for approximately 6 weeks but should be active, with a goal of ambulation within 8 h of surgery and three times daily.

Take-Home Messages
- A laparoscopic approach is a safe and feasible option for repair of incarcerated hernias.
- For inguinal hernias, a transperitoneal approach, rather than extraperitoneal approach, is preferred due to the ability to inspect the bowel.
- Incarcerated hernias without full-thickness bowel injury or contamination may be repaired with synthetic mesh. In hernia repairs with concern for necrosis or injury to the bowel requiring resection, primary repair or placement of biologic mesh should be considered.
- When safe and feasible, delay the repair of large ventral hernias to actively address modifiable patient risk factors (such as tobacco cessation, weight loss, and blood glucose control) for optimal control of wound infection and recurrence rates.

References

1. Poulose BK, Shelton J, Phillips S, et al. Epidemiology and cost of ventral hernia repair: making the case for hernia research. Hernia. 2012;16(2):179–83. doi:10.1007/s10029-011-0879-9.
2. Beadles CA, Meagher AD, Charles AG. Trends in emergent hernia repair in the United States. JAMA Surg. 2015;150(3):194–200. doi:10.1001/jamasurg.2014.1242.
3. Kingsnorth A, LeBlanc K. Hernias: inguinal and incisional. Lancet (London, England). 2003;362(9395):1561–71. doi:10.1016/S0140-6736(03)14746-0.
4. Fitzgibbons RJ, Cemaj S, Quinn TH. Abdominal wall hernias. In: Mulholland M, editor. Greenfield's surgery scientific principles and practice. 11th ed. Philadelphia: Lippincott; 2011.
5. Novitsky YW, Orenstein SB. Effect of patient and hospital characteristics on outcomes of elective ventral hernia repair in the United States. Hernia. 2013;17(5):639–45. doi:10.1007/s10029-013-1088-5.
6. Hornby ST, McDermott FD, Coleman M, et al. Female gender and diabetes mellitus increase the risk of recurrence after laparoscopic incisional hernia repair. Ann R Coll Surg Engl. 2015;97(2):115–9. doi:10.1308/003588414X14055925058751.
7. Colavita PD, Zemlyak AY, Burton PV, Dacey KT, Walters AL, Lincourt AE, Tsirline VE, Kercher KW, Heniford BT. The expansive cost of wound infections after ventral hernia repair. Washington, DC: American College of Surgeons; 2013.
8. Fitzgibbons RJ, Giobbie-Hurder A, Gibbs JO, et al. Watchful waiting vs repair of inguinal hernia in minimally symptomatic men: a randomized clinical trial. JAMA. 2006;295(3):285–92. doi:10.1001/jama.295.3.285.
9. Fitzgibbons RJ, Ramanan B, Arya S, et al. Long-term results of a randomized controlled trial of a nonoperative strategy (watchful waiting) for men with minimally symptomatic inguinal hernias. Ann Surg. 2013;258(3):508–15. doi:10.1097/SLA.0b013e3182a19725.
10. Belyansky I, Tsirline VB, Klima DA, Walters AL, Lincourt AE, Heniford BT. Prospective, comparative study of postoperative quality of life in TEP, TAPP, and modified Lichtenstein repairs. Ann Surg. 2011;254(5):709–15. doi:10.1097/SLA.0b013e3182359d07.
11. Tsirline VB, Colavita PD, Belyansky I, Zemlyak AY, Lincourt AE, Heniford BT. Preoperative pain is the strongest predictor of postoperative pain and diminished quality of life after ventral hernia repair. Am Surg 2013;79(8):829–836. http://www.ncbi.nlm.nih.gov/pubmed/23896254. Accessed 30 Oct 2016.
12. Rosenberg J, Bisgaard T, Kehlet H, et al. Danish hernia database recommendations for the management of inguinal and femoral hernia in adults. Dan Med Bull 2011;58(2):C4243. http://www.ncbi.nlm.nih.gov/pubmed/21299930. Accessed 13 June 2016.
13. Altom LK, Snyder CW, Gray SH, Graham LA, Vick CC, Hawn MT. Outcomes of emergent incisional hernia repair. Am Surg 2011;77(8):971–976. http://www.ncbi.nlm.nih.gov/pubmed/21944508. Accessed 9 July 2016.
14. Landau O, Kyzer S. Emergent laparoscopic repair of incarcerated incisional and ventral hernia. Surg Endosc. 2004;18(9):1374–6. doi:10.1007/s00464-003-9116-7.
15. Yang GPC, Chan CTY, Lai ECH, Chan OCY, Tang CN, Li MKW. Laparoscopic versus open repair for strangulated groin hernias: 188 cases over 4 years. Asian J Endosc Surg. 2012;5(3):131–7. doi:10.1111/j.1758-5910.2012.00138.x.
16. Chang P. Chapter 39: Emergent surgical management of ventral hernias. In: Novitsky YW, editor, Hernia surgery: current principles. 1st ed. Cleveland; Springer Publishing. 2016. p. 401–8.
17. Chen T, Zhang Y, Wang H, et al. Emergency inguinal hernia repair under local anesthesia: a 5-year experience in a teaching hospital. BMC Anesthesiol. 2016;16(1):17. doi:10.1186/s12871-016-0185-2.
18. Earle D, Roth S, Saber A, et al. SAGES guidelines for laparoscopic ventral hernia repair. 2014. http://www.sages.org/publications/guidelines/guidelines-for-laparoscopic-ventral-hernia-repair/.

19. Ferzli G, Shapiro K, Chaudry G, Patel S. Laparoscopic extraperitoneal approach to acutely incarcerated inguinal hernia. Surg Endosc. 2004;18(2):228–31. doi:10.1007/s00464-003-8185-y.
20. Huerta S, Pham T, Foster S, Livingston EH, Dineen S. Outcomes of emergent inguinal hernia repair in veteran octogenarians. Am Surg 2014;80(5):479–483. http://www.ncbi.nlm.nih.gov/pubmed/24887727. Accessed 9 July 2016.
21. Martínez-Serrano MA, Pereira JA, Sancho JJ, et al. Risk of death after emergency repair of abdominal wall hernias. Still waiting for improvement. Langenbeck's Arch Surg (Dtsch Gesellschaft für Chir). 2010;395(5):551–6. doi:10.1007/s00423-009-0515-7.
22. Colavita PD, Tsirline VB, Belyansky I, et al. Prospective, long-term comparison of quality of life in laparoscopic versus open ventral hernia repair. Ann Surg. 2012;256(5):714–23. doi:10.1097/SLA.0b013e3182734130.

Further Reading

1. Altom LK, Snyder CW, Gray SH, Graham LA, Vick CC, Hawn MT. Outcomes of emergent incisional hernia repair. Am Surgeon. 2011;77(8):971–6.
2. Chang P. Chapter 39: Emergent surgical management of ventral hernias. In: Novitsky YW, editor. Hernia surgery: current principles. Cleveland: Springer Publishing; 2016.
3. Jagad RB, Shah J, Patel GR. The laparoscopic transperitoneal approach for irreducible inguinal hernias: perioperative outcome in four patients. J Minim Access Surg. 2009;5(2):31–4.
4. Landau O, Kyzer S. Emergent laparoscopic repair of incarcerated incisional and ventral hernia. Surg Endosc. 2014;18(9):1374–6.
5. Yeh DD, Alam HB. Hernia emergencies. Surg Clin N Am. 2014;94(1):97–130.

Lee L. Swanström and Kristin Beard

Introduction

Hiatal hernia is a condition in which the esophageal hiatus of the diaphragm is sufficiently enlarged to allow for the migration of abdominal contents into the posterior mediastinum and can be associated with compressive symptoms or torsion. The incidence is estimated to be between 10% and 60% of the population. Giant hiatal hernias rarely present before age 50, but become more prevalent in older populations. Familial predisposition, particularly to PEH, has been noted, but the mechanism for inheritance is not yet clear. The pathophysiology of hiatal hernia is incompletely understood and likely multifactorial. It is usually acquired, though some developmental abnormalities have been proposed. Altered collagen metabolism and extracellular matrix derangements have been implicated in breakdown of the diaphragmatic tissues. Excessive intra-abdominal pressure and negative intrathoracic pressure add further stress to the diaphragm, especially in the setting of chronic cough, obesity, pregnancy, or chronic constipation. Laxity and attenuation of the diaphragmatic crura, associated ligaments, and peritoneal attachments result in an enlarged hiatus. A peritoneal sac develops. The gastric fundus, gastroesophageal junction (GEJ), and sometimes other organs push up into the mediastinal sac to varying degrees (Fig. 4.1). Over time, foreshortening and fibrosis of the esophagus, opening of the angle of His, and associated gastroesophageal reflux disease (GERD) can all develop.

Hiatal hernias are anatomically characterized. The most common hernia is a small type I sliding hernia. These hiatal hernias are at minimal risk of incarceration. In isolation, a small type I hiatal hernia does not require repair, except with a concomitant anti-reflux procedure in the setting of objective evidence of GERD. Surgical repair is indicated for symptomatic paraesophageal hernia (PEH) type II–IV. These represent only 5–10% of all hiatal hernias (Fig. 4.2). A PEH is termed "giant" if greater than 30–50% of the stomach is above the diaphragm or simply "intrathoracic stomach" when the majority of the stomach is in the chest. Acute incarceration, volvulus, and strangulation are the dreaded complications of paraesophageal hernia, though NSQIP data from 2005 to 2012 found that only 3.5% of all PEH repairs were emergent [1]. Although rare, acute incarceration can be life threatening, potentially leading to hemorrhage, ischemia, or perforation.

Preoperative Diagnosis

Incidental vs Acute

In 1967, Skinner published a 29% mortality rate associated with nonoperative management of symptomatic paraesophageal hernia [2]. For decades, elective repair of all paraesophageal hernias was recommended based on this report. Throughout the years, as surgical techniques and medical management improved, the strategy for managing PEH patients evolved. A well-known Markov analysis released in 2002 shifted the paradigm, concluding that minimally symptomatic patients ought to be managed with watchful waiting, as the risk of requiring emergent repair and associated mortality was outweighed by the mortality rate of elective repair [3]. This was based on published mortality rates of up to 17% with emergency repair, a 1.1% risk per year of requiring emergency repair in asymptomatic patients. This extrapolated to an 18% mortality risk for emergent repair in patients 65 years or older, compared to published 1% mortality risk of elective surgery. However, a more recent review of 10,656 NSQIP patients found only a 5.5% mortality rate for all

L.L. Swanström, MD (✉)
Oregon Health and Sciences University, Portland, OR, USA

IHU-Strasbourg, Strasbourg, France
e-mail: lswanstrom@gmail.com

K. Beard, MD
Portland Providence Hospital, Providence Cancer Center, Portland, OR, USA
e-mail: Kristin.wilson.beard@gmail.com

© Springer International Publishing AG 2018
K.A. Khwaja, J.J. Diaz (eds.), *Minimally Invasive Acute Care Surgery*, https://doi.org/10.1007/978-3-319-64723-4_4

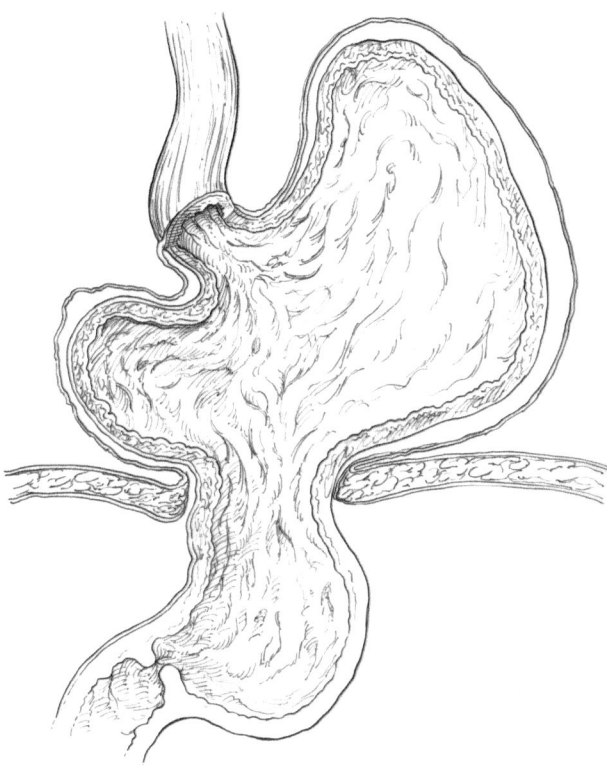

Fig. 4.1 Paraesophageal hernias are a result of attenuation of the phrenoesophageal ligament and herniation of the peritoneal sac and lesser sac into the mediastinum

emergency PEH repairs and 0.46% rate of mortality for laparoscopic elective repairs [4]. As technique and outcomes for repair continue to improve, some experts are beginning to consider repair of minimally symptomatic patients (i.e., those with GERD alone) given the relative safety in the hands of experienced laparoscopic surgeons [5].

Symptomatic paraesophageal hernia should trigger consideration of repair, whether elective or acute. While nonspecific, intermittent dysphagia, regurgitation, chest or epigastric pain radiating to the back, shortness of breath, and palpitations (when cardiac and other causes have been ruled out) are some presenting symptoms for intermittent obstruction or volvulus of the hernia. Intractable symptoms suggest acute incarceration with strangulation and require admission, resuscitation, and medical optimization in preparation for urgent surgical repair. Borchardt's classic triad of epigastric pain, retching without vomiting, and inability to pass a nasogastric tube is not always present, nor required for diagnosis.

Physical Examination and Laboratory Tests

The examination of the patient with an acutely incarcerated PEH is usually nonspecific and unrevealing, lacking signifi-
cant physical exam findings unless perforation or other complication has occurred. Laboratory values are nonspecific as well, but anemia related to acute hemorrhage or chronic iron deficiency from mucosal injury is present in about one third of the cases. Signs of sepsis may be identified in the case of perforation and are used to guide resuscitation and timing of operative intervention. Multisystem organ dysfunction is ominous, particularly in the frail, elderly, or comorbid patient.

Imaging Tests

Chest radiography may identify a retrocardiac shadow or air-fluid level. Free intraperitoneal air, pneumothorax, or pleural effusion are menacing signs and should prompt urgent surgical intervention. If the diagnosis is in question, a contrast esophagram is a useful study for an elective evaluation, but in the urgent situation, a CT of the chest and abdomen is more appropriate. In the acute setting, there is no indication to obtain pH or manometry studies. However, most admissions and ED workups for PEH are in stable patients without acute incarceration, and these patients can complete the physiologic workup in an outpatient setting. Manometry can further identify the size of a hernia, document outflow obstruction or esophageal dysmotility, and may guide the surgeon's choice of fundoplication. Manometry catheter placement may be difficult due to anatomic factors. Even if a full study is unobtainable, information about the esophageal body (length and function) is useful. Fundoplication is routinely performed with PEH repair, as 60% of patients will have GERD symptoms and 20–40% will have positive pH study if repaired without a fundoplication. Therefore, preoperative pH testing is not mandatory for type II–IV PEH as it does not alter the surgical management. Endoscopy should be performed as a routine part of the preoperative and intraoperative evaluation of paraesophageal hernia. Endoscopy is critical to evaluate for esophagitis or stricture, hemorrhage, mucosal ischemia, or ulceration and is useful to evaluate the size and type of the hernia and identify volvulus.

Management

Preoperative Preparation

For acutely incarcerated and obstructed PEH, the patient should be admitted and optimized for surgical exploration. Nasogastric tube placement or endoscopy with decompression should be attempted. Resuscitation followed by rapid progression to the operating room is recommended. Early intervention may help to speed recovery and reduce risk of complications, such as venous thromboembolism or pulmo-

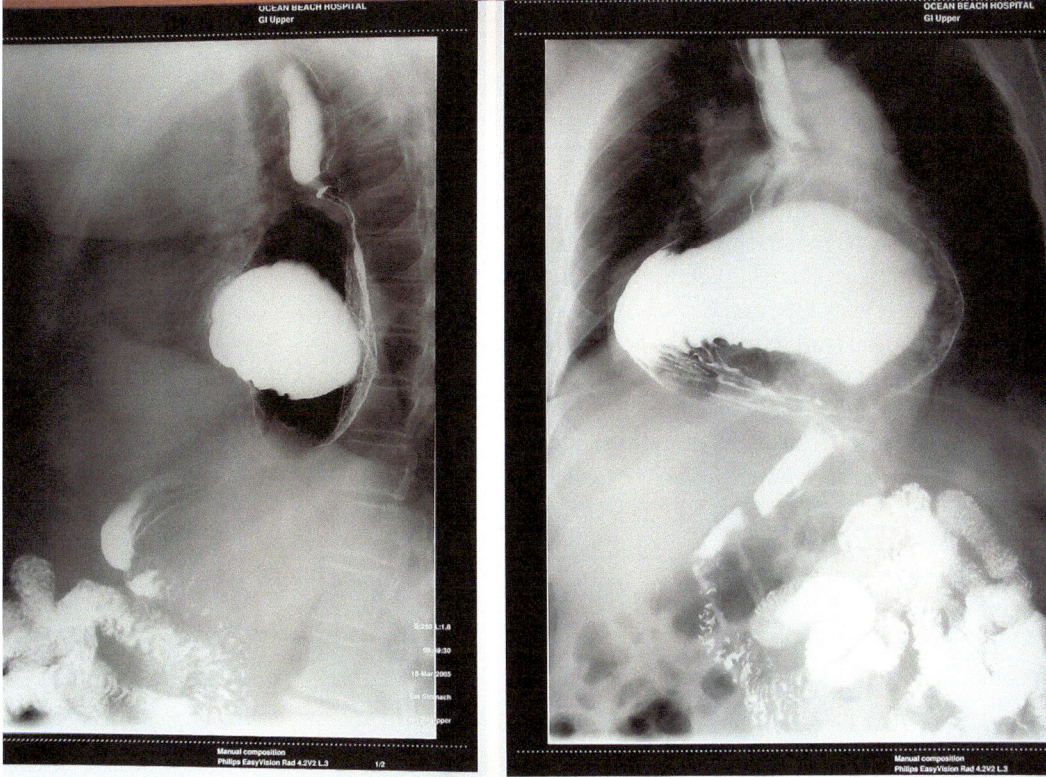

Fig. 4.2   Paraesophageal hernias are classified as type II, III, or IV

nary edema [6]. A Foley catheter is placed to guide resuscitation. Preoperative prophylactic antibiotics are given routinely, broad spectrum if there are signs of sepsis. A type and crossmatch is collected especially in cases with acute GI bleeding.

Surgical principles include complete reduction of the stomach and associated organs, excision of the hernia sac, mediastinal dissection and assessment of esophageal length, repair of the diaphragmatic hiatus, maintenance of the stomach below the diaphragm via fundoplication, or gastropexy with a gastrostomy tube. The laparoscopic approach has become the preferred approach in the elective setting and is usually feasible in the emergent setting in experienced hands though it is an advanced case and should have a low threshold for conversion to open. Challenges of the laparoscopic approach include management of the large hernia sac and mobilization of a foreshortened esophagus. The traditional approach by thoracotomy has the benefit of generous exposure of the hernia sac and easier angles for an esophageal lengthening procedure if it is required. The disadvantage of thoracotomy is that it leaves the surgeon blind to the abdomen where volvulus may persist; it leads to more pain, more pulmonary complications, and longer hospital stay. Thoracoscopic repair is not generally performed due to lack of space to work in the left chest. Laparotomy can be per-

formed as well and facilitates the creation of the fundoplication; however, the downside of laparotomy is diminished visualization of the hiatus and mediastinum, particularly in the obese patient. Open surgery is preferred when the patient is unstable despite resuscitative efforts and will not tolerate laparoscopy or the surgeon lacks advanced laparoscopic experience. Relative indications may include frank peritonitis with significant spillage or reoperative upper abdomen. The usual tenets for converting to an open procedure apply, such as inability to make safe progress, hemorrhage that cannot be controlled laparoscopically, or uncorrectable hemodynamic instability due to insufflation pressure effects on venous return. Rarely both abdominal and thoracic access may be required if there is significant spillage into the chest or inability to reduce the hernia contents safely through the transabdominal approach.

Considerations

Key points of the laparoscopic surgery are:

- Reduction of the hernia sac
- Mobilization of the mediastinal esophagus
- Collis gastroplasty if needed
- Reinforced repair of the hiatus
- Tailored fundoplication

The surgeon must always consider the overall condition of the patient, and in the case of persistent instability, a damage control operation can be performed. The tissue integrity of the stomach, esophagus, duodenum, and any other herniated organs must be assessed. Perforations or ischemic tissue that does not reperfuse after hernia reduction must be identified and managed with drainage, repair, or formal resection. If a damage control strategy is required, then once the hernia is reduced, necrotic tissue debrided, and viscus closed, a simple gastrostomy tube may be placed to pexy the stomach to the abdominal wall to reduce the hernia and allow decompression. In rare cases, gastric or esophageal resection is needed and should be accompanied by feeding access and a proximal diversion (spit fistula). Reconstruction can then be scheduled in a delayed fashion to allow recovery.

General Approach to Repair (Technical Considerations) [7]

The patient is positioned on an orthopedic OR table with the legs split, secured, and supported with footboards and with both arms out. The operating surgeon works from the patient's left side, with an assistant to manage the camera and retract position between the patient's feet. An incision is made in the left upper quadrant, at about the midpoint between the costal margin in the midclavicular line and the umbilicus. A Veress needle is used for insufflation, and a 10 mm camera trocar is placed. A 10 mm 45-degree high-definition laparoscope is introduced and will be controlled by the assistant's right hand. The patient is placed in steep reverse Trendelenburg. A 5 mm trocar is placed laterally, just below the left costal margin for the surgeon's right hand. A 5 mm trocar is placed for the assistant's left hand, directly lateral to the camera port just to the right of midline. A 5 mm trocar is placed superior to this trocar and just inferior to the costal margin and used for a serpentine liver retractor. The left lobe is elevated and retracted to the right away from the hiatus and secured to a table-mounted retractor holder, positioned at the patient's right axilla. Finally, a 5 mm trocar for the surgeon's left hand is placed in the subxiphoid area (Fig. 4.3).

The general tenant of reducing giant hiatal hernias laparoscopically should be conceptualized as a process of reducing the bilobar (anterior, peritoneal and posterior, or lesser sac) hernia sac, as opposed to reducing the contents of the sac. The mediastinal hernia sac is grasped within the mediastinum at the 12 o'clock position, and the sack is partially inverted into the abdomen. Though tempting, grabbing the stomach, omentum, or other herniated viscus should be avoided. Traction on these structures – working against the laparoscopic insufflation pressure – can easily result in tears, particularly if there is a degree of ischemia. The only exception is a tightly incarcerated hernia allowing no access to the

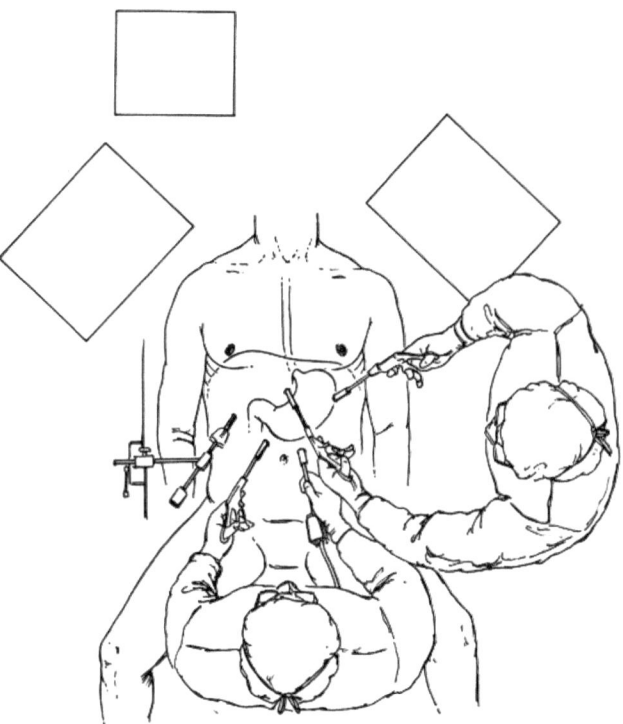

Fig. 4.3 A typical patient and trocar position for PEH repair (Reprinted with permission from Ref. [17])

hernia sac. In this case, gentle traction and lysis of adhesions should be performed until the omentum and small bowel/colon can be reduced and allow access to the hernia sac. Likewise, we believe approaching the gastrohepatic ligament first, as in a typical Nissen fundoplication, is not a good idea as the left gastric artery and other neural-vascular structures along the lesser curve herniate across the right crus and into the mediastinum and might be accidently injured. The sac (elongated phrenoesophageal ligament) is opened at the hiatal apex with ultrasonic shears. Blunt dissection should identify the proper plane, which should be bloodless. A combination of blunt sweeping and ultrasonic dissection, while at the same time detaching the sac from the rim of the hiatus, will slowly allow the mediastinal hernia sac (and its contents) to be reduced into the abdomen. The process of reducing the contents becomes easier as the insufflation pressure switches from pushing the hernia sac back into the mediastinum to one where it starts pushing the sac into the abdomen. Once the left side of the mediastinal hernia sac is reduced, the gastrohepatic ligament can be opened to expose the right crus. The right side of the anterior and posterior sacs is reduced/detached similar to the left side. Sac dissection should continue well onto the decussation of the crura. At this point – and without putting traction on the stomach – the hernia and its contents have been reduced.

It is next universally necessary to mobilize the mediastinal esophagus. Anterior and posterior vagus nerves are identified and preserved. While the assistant retracts the GEJ caudally while pulling on the hernia sac, the surgeon progressively mobilizes the esophagus by progressive blunt dissection and ultrasonic/bipolar dissection. In a large hiatal hernia, this dissection is relatively easy to continue until the level of the carina or azygos (Fig. 4.4). The goal of this mobilization is to achieve 2.5–3 cm of tension-free intra-abdominal esophageal length (Fig. 4.5). It is frequently necessary to identify the true GEJ and insure that the esophagus has been adequately mobilized, by performing intraoperative endoscopy and transillumination of the GEJ. In 2–6% of the cases, in spite of extensive esophageal mobilization, the GEJ may not reach the abdomen. This true, intrinsic short esophagus may be due to esophagitis, stricture, or chronic fibrosis; regardless, it must be addressed, or either the fundoplication will be placed on the stomach or the repair will be under axial tension and have an extremely high recurrence rate [8]. Dividing one or both vagus nerves to achieve several centimeters of additional length has been proposed. A low rate of subsequent gastroparesis or dumping syndrome is reported [9]. We prefer to preserve the vagus nerves whenever possible and perform a Collis gastroplasty when additional esophageal length is required. Two different techniques for Collis

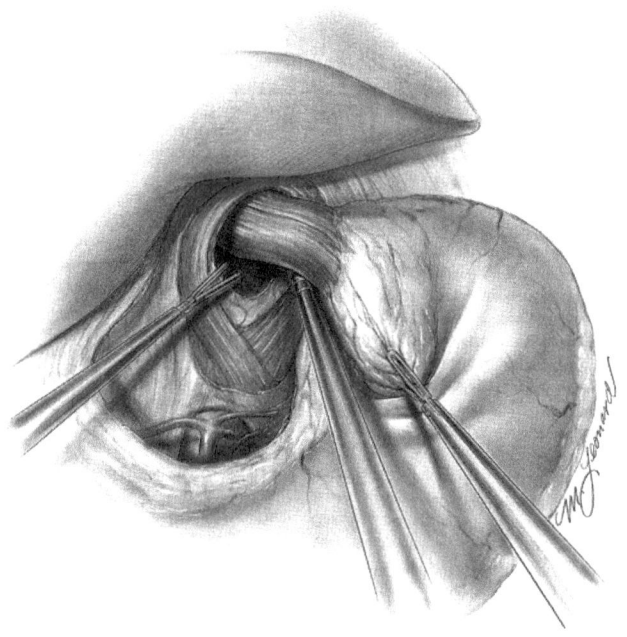

Fig. 4.5 The end goal of mediastinal dissection is 2.5–3 cm of tension-free intra-abdominal esophageal length (Reprinted with permission from Ref. [17])

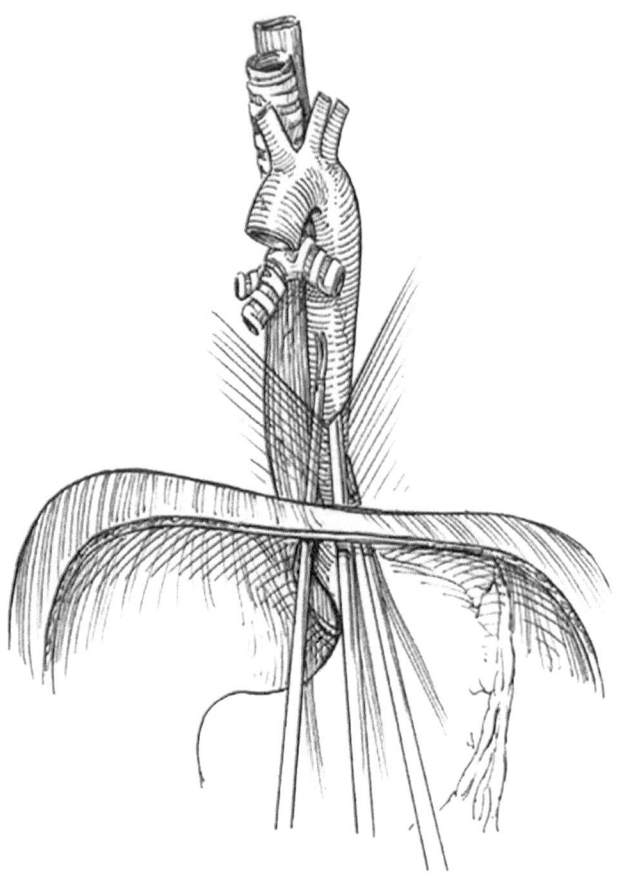

Fig. 4.4 High, transmediastinal esophageal dissection is almost always required for giant PEH (Reprinted with permission from Ref. [17])

gastroplasty are in common use: either a left transthoracic, transmediastinal single fire staple technique, which replicates a traditional open procedure, or a newer procedure that laparoscopically resects the fundus of the stomach to add length to the esophagus (wedge fundectomy) [10, 11] (Fig. 4.6a, b). Problems with Collis gastroplasty include higher leak rate, acid-secreting mucosa in the neoesophagus, altered motility, stenosis, the development of diverticulum, and difficulty of revision.

During mediastinal hernia sac reduction or esophageal mobilization, particularly in cases with extensive fibrosis or inflammation, the mediastinal pleura may be unavoidably entered, and capnothorax results. If pleural injury occurs, do not panic. Communicate with your anesthesiologist. They should be able to manage any changes in CO_2 or ventilation with the addition of positive end-expiratory pressure to re-expand the lung and hyperventilation to control the pCO_2. Hypotension due to tension physiology is extremely rare. If pleura is breached, it is important to remember it is a capnothorax which (1) rapidly absorbs and (2) is under the surgeon's control. A laparoscopic suction can be used to evacuate the CO_2 from the intrapleural space and the abdomen desufflated if hemodynamic problems arise. If there are no hemodynamic changes, the capnothorax can safely be ignored. At the end of the procedure, repeated intrapleural and mediastinal surgical suctioning, with the patient head down during several Valsalva maneuvers, can be performed, but residual CO_2 is typically resorbed in a few hours. A chest

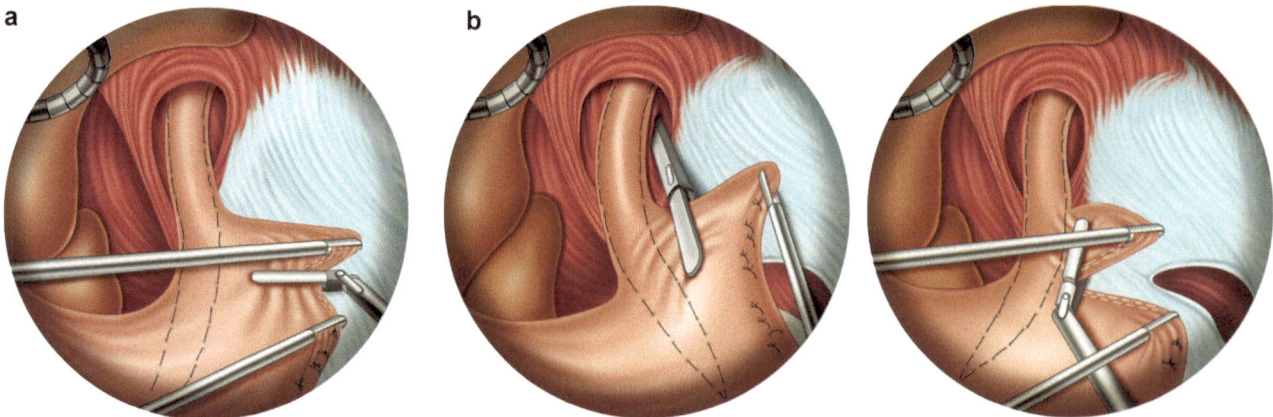

Fig. 4.6 (**a**) Transthoracic single staple fire method of Collis gastroplasty. (**bi**) and (**bii**) Wedge fundectomy completely laparoscopic Collis technique (Reprinted with permission from Ref. [17])

tube is almost never required for capnothorax unless associated with gross contamination from a perforated viscus.

Diaphragmatic closure. When adequate esophageal length is obtained, the crural defect is closed. It is typical to close the hiatus posteriorly, but important not to kink the distal esophagus posteriorly. Anterior closure sutures are acceptable and sometimes needed [12]. Unless there is contamination, we incorporate a biologic mesh simultaneously with the posterior crural closure. We use three horizontal mattress sutures of 0 Ethibond with Teflon pledgets placed through the mesh and then the left and right crura (Fig. 4.7). This results in the mesh being tightly applied to the closure to improve incorporation. The sutures are tied extracorporeally using either a knot pusher or a Ti-Knot device according to the surgeon's preference. Others describe primary crural closure and subsequent onlay mesh with sutures, tacks (not recommended due to hemopericardium reports), or glue. When

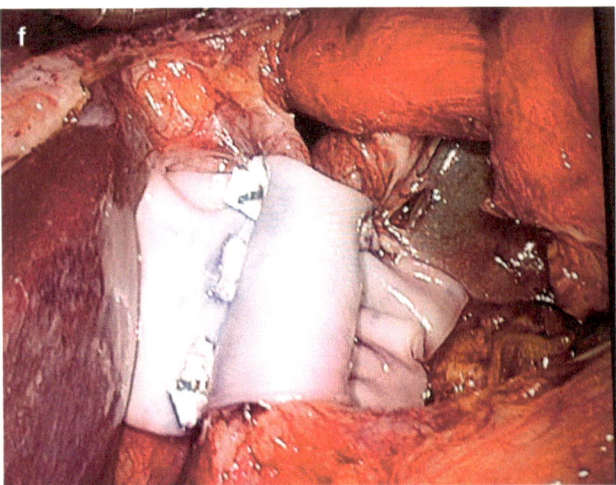

Fig. 4.7 Posterior hiatal closure using pledgeted horizontal mattress sutures and incorporating biologic mesh (Reprinted with permission from Ref. [17])

the gap is too large or the crura too fibrotic to close without undo tension, a single or bilateral relaxing incision may be used to aid in medialization (Fig. 4.8). The resulting diaphragmatic defect is closed with permanent bridging mesh, placed remotely well from the esophagus.

The use of either permanent or biologic mesh to supplement primary repair remains controversial. There is evidence for short-term reduction of recurrence with biologic mesh placement, though recurrence rates are still near 50% in longer-term follow-up [13]. Most recurrences are minimally symptomatic, and only 3–5% go on to require revision [16]. Permanent mesh has been shown to decrease recurrence rates in randomized studies [14] but at the price of potential erosion [15], and it is almost never indicated in an acute strangulation/perforation.

Anti-reflux Procedure

It is typical to add a fundoplication in conjunction with a laparoscopic paraesophageal hernia repair. Aside from questions regarding the possibility of postoperative reflux, the fundoplication is felt to further anchor the stomach in the peritoneal cavity and buttress the diaphragmatic repair. If preoperative manometry is normal, standard Nissen fundoplication is employed. However, if preoperative body motility is diminished as noted by less than 60–70% peristalsis, DECA <25, or weak DCI, if preoperative manometry could not be obtained, or if dysphagia was a significant preoperative symptom, we prefer to perform a Toupet fundoplication. Once again, in damage control situations, with an unstable patient, the fundoplication should be skipped and only hiatal closure quickly performed, and consideration can be given to a gastropexy.

Feeding Access

In a horrendous case with perforation, hemorrhage, or poor tissue quality, alternative feeding access should be consid-

Fig. 4.8 Diaphragm relaxing incisions can be made in either right or left diaphragm and subsequently covered with a mesh (Reprinted with permission from Ref. [17])

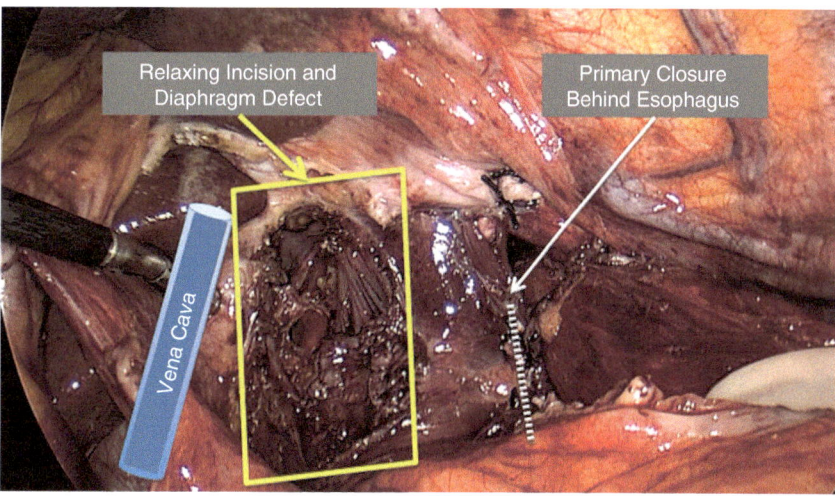

ered. A gastrostomy can be placed to pexy, decompress, and eventually feed the stomach, and/or a jejunostomy can be placed to feed distal to the affected area. If no fundoplication was performed, a jejunostomy would be a preferable feeding access to avoid aspiration from reflux.

Procedure Completion

At least one drain is placed through the crural opening into the mediastinum primarily to ablate the dead space and minimize seroma formation; more drains can be placed and positioned depending on other areas of concern. Finally, an endoscopy is performed to evaluate the repair and ensure the fundoplication appears appropriate, the SCJ is below the fundoplication, and a leak insufflation test can be performed for any problem areas.

Postoperative Concerns

Postoperatively, ICU care may be required in the acute setting for hemodynamic or pulmonary concerns, but most elective or semi-urgent cases will not require critical care. The patient is kept NPO overnight. An upper gastrointestinal (UGI) contrast study is completed the morning after surgery if the patient is otherwise stable. Drain amylase is followed for at least one check postoperatively. If no signs of leak, gastroesophageal junction obstruction, or gastric ileus, then a liquid diet and crushed/liquid meds are started and progressed to full liquids. A diet of liquid or puree is kept for 2 weeks post-op. In-office follow-up is routine at 1 month. At 1 year repeat studies are performed, including UGI to evaluate anatomy and recurrence, pH, and manometry to assess the integrity of esophageal function and the anti-reflux barrier. Endoscopy is used selectively for patients who have specific symptoms or findings on the remaining testing.

Small recurrences are not uncommonly seen – particularly after 5 years. As these are usually asymptomatic, no specific treatment is required, but the patients may benefit from closer follow-up [16].

Take-Home Messages
1. Strangulation or acute obstructive incarceration of giant PEH is not as common as once thought.
2. Strangulation or acute obstructive incarceration of giant PEH is potentially lethal and should be addressed emergently or during admission depending on the status of the patient.
3. Preoperative endoscopy may allow detorsion and convert an emergent case to an urgent one.
4. If the team has a high level of skill and experience, a laparoscopic attempt at reduction and repair of acute PEH is reasonable. If not, an open transthoracic repair should be performed even though this is a more morbid and patient-unfriendly approach.
5. Laparoscopic repair of giant PEH involves the following steps: mediastinal sac reduction, atraumatic detachment of phrenoesophageal ligament from the crural rim, extensive mediastinal dissection of the esophagus (until 2.5–3 cm of intra-abdominal esophagus is obtained.), reinforced crural closure, and fundoplication.
6. If crura cannot be closed primarily, diaphragmatic relaxing incision is probably the best option.
7. A Collis gastroplasty may be needed if there is intrinsic esophageal shortening.

Key References

1. Augustin T, Schneider E, Alaedeen D, Kroh M, Aminian A, Reznick D, Walsh M, Brethauer S. Emergent surgery does not independently predict 30-day mortality after paraesophageal hernia repair: results from the ACS NSQIP database. J Gastrointest Surg. 2015 Dec;19(12):2097–104.
2. Ellis FH Jr. Esophageal hiatal hernia. N Engl J Med. 1972;287(13):646–9.
3. Stylopoulos N, Gazelle GS, Rattner DW. Paraesophageal hernias: operation or observation? Ann Surg. 2002;236:492–500. discussion 500–501.
4. Jassim H, Seligman JT, Frelich M, Goldblatt M, Kastenmeier A, Wallace J, Zhao HS, Szabo A, Gould JC. A population-based analysis of emergent versus elective paraesophageal hernia repair using the Nationwide inpatient sample. Surg Endosc. 2014;28(12):3473–8. doi:10.1007/s00464-014-3626-3. Epub 2014 Jun 18.
5. Mungo B, Molena D, Stem M, Feinberg RL, Lidor AO. Thirty-day outcomes of paraesophageal hernia repair using the NSQIP database: should laparoscopy be the standard of care? J Am Coll Surg. 2014;219(2):229–36.
6. Bhayani NH, Kurian AA, Sharata AM, Reavis KM, Dunst CM, Swanstrom LL. Wait only to resuscitate: early surgery for acutely presenting paraesophageal hernias yields better outcomes. Surg Endosc. 2013;27(1):267–71.
7. DeMeester SR. Laparoscopic paraesophageal hernia repair: critical steps and adjunct techniques to minimize recurrence. Surg Laparosc Endosc Percutan Tech. 2013;23(5):429–35.
8. Gastal OL, Hagen JA, Peters JH, et al. Short esophagus: analysis of predictors and clinical implications. Arch Surg. 1999;134:633–6; discussion 7–8.
9. Oelschlager BK, Yamamoto K, Woltman T, Pellegrini C. Vagotomy during hiatal hernia repair: a benign esophageal lengthening procedure. J Gastrointest Surg. 2008;12(7):1155–62. doi:10.1007/s11605-008-0520-0. Epub 2008 May 8.
10. Horvath KD, Swanstrom LL, Jobe BA. The short esophagus: pathophysiology, incidence, presentation, and treatment in the era of laparoscopic Antireflux surgery. Ann Surg. 2000;232(5):630–40.
11. Terry ML, Vernon A, Hunter JG. Stapled-wedge Collis gastroplasty for the shortened esophagus. Am J Surg. 2004;188:195–9.
12. Watson DI, Jamieson GG, Devitt PG, Kennedy JA, Ellis T, Ackroyd R, Lafullarde T, Game PA. A prospective randomized trial of laparoscopic Nissen fundoplication with anterior vs posterior hiatal repair. Arch Surg. 2001;136(7):745–51.
13. Oelschlager BK, Pellegrini CA, Hunter JG, et al. Biologic prosthesis to prevent recurrence after laparoscopic para-esophageal hernia repair: long-term follow-up from a multi-center, prospective, randomized trial. J Am Coll Surg. 2011;213:461–8.
14. Müller-Stich BP, Kenngott HG, Gondan M, Stock C, Linke GR, Fritz F, Nickel F, Diener MK, Gutt CN, Wente M, Büchler MW, Fischer L. Use of mesh in laparoscopic paraesophageal hernia repair: a meta-analysis and risk-benefit analysis. PLoS One. 2015;10(10):e0139547. doi:10.1371/journal.pone.0139547. Review. Erratum in: PLoS One. 2017 Feb 3;12 (2):e0171865.
15. Stadlhuber RJ, Sherif AE, Mittal SK, et al. Mesh complications after prosthetic reinforcement of hiatal closure: a 28-case series. Surg Endosc. 2009;23:1219–26.
16. Oelschlager BK, Petersen RP, Brunt LM, et al. Laparoscopic para-esophageal hernia repair: defining long-term clinical and anatomic outcomes. J Gastrointest Surg. 2012;16:453–9.
17. Swanstrom LL, Dunst CM. Antireflux surgery. New York: Springer; 2015.

Mark D. Kligman

Introduction

Over the last three decades, bariatric surgery has gained acceptance as a primary treatment for morbid obesity. This is largely due to the accumulating evidence demonstrating that surgical weight loss results in durable improvement in obesity-related comorbidities, as well as improved surgical morbidity and mortality. As a result, the number of bariatric surgery procedures has increased rapidly, with about 193,000 operations performed in 2014. The acute care surgeon will encounter these patients with increasing frequency and must have a working knowledge regarding the evaluation and management of bariatric surgery complications.

Bariatric operations can be classified as restrictive, malabsorptive, or combined procedures. The mainstay bariatric procedures are sleeve gastrectomy, gastric bypass, adjustable gastric band, and biliopancreatic diversion with duodenal switch (Fig. 5.1). Sleeve gastrectomy, in which the greater curvature of the stomach is resected over a 34–40 French bougie to create a lesser curvature tube, is currently the most popular procedure. The primary advantages of this restrictive operation are its technical simplicity and paucity of late complications. Roux-en-Y gastric bypass, once the "gold standard" operation, is now the second most common operation. This operation creates a 15–30 mL gastric pouch, drained by a 75–150 cm Roux limb through a 10–15 mm gastrojejunostomy. The bypassed stomach (gastric remnant) is drained by the biliopancreatic limb that joins the Roux limb to form the common channel. This operation is primarily restrictive, combined with limited malabsorption determined by the length of the Roux limb. Adjustable gastric banding, once performed commonly, is now waning in popularity. The band, which has an inflatable balloon along its inner surface, is positioned just below the gastroesophageal junction, creating a small gastric pouch cephalad. Adjusting the balloon volume with sterile water via the subcutaneous port optimizes restriction. However, the simplicity of the procedure is offset by a high reoperation rate for mechanical complications. Biliopancreatic diversion with duodenal switch (BPD-DS) is a malabsorptive procedure. This is an uncommon operation that provides excellent weight loss and comorbidity improvement. In BPD-DS, sleeve gastrectomy forms the proximal operation. The duodenum is divided distal to the duodenal bulb and anastomosed to the divided end of the distal 200–300 cm of the small intestine. All remaining proximal intestine forms the biliopancreatic limb, which is anastomosed to the common channel 50–150 cm proximal to the ileocecal valve. The management of complications of BPD-DS and other uncommon operations is beyond the scope of this discussion.

A list of common operative complications for the three most common bariatric surgery procedures is shown in Table 5.1. Most bariatric surgery complications encountered by the acute care surgeon can be categorized as either leaks or obstructions. The exception is marginal ulcer, a complication of gastric bypass, which has a varied presentation. While principles of management are independent of the treatment method, a well-prepared acute care surgeon can manage many of these complications using endoscopic or laparoscopic techniques.

General Operative Considerations

The decision to use a laparoscopic approach for the management of bariatric surgery complications is based on the surgeon's experience and on patient-related factors. The surgeon's comfort with laparoscopic suturing is the primary determinant of the surgical approach. Assistive suturing devices can be used in many instances, but surgeons should be prepared to convert to laparotomy if these devices prove inadequate for the clinical situation. In addition, complex reconstructions (i.e., operations requiring resection and re-anastomosis) are particularly challenging, due to the

M.D. Kligman, M.D. (✉)
Assistant Professor, Director, Department of Surgery, Center for Weight Management & Wellness, University of Maryland School of Medicine, 29 South Greene Street, Suite 105, Baltimore, MD 21201, USA
e-mail: mkligman@smail.umaryland.edu

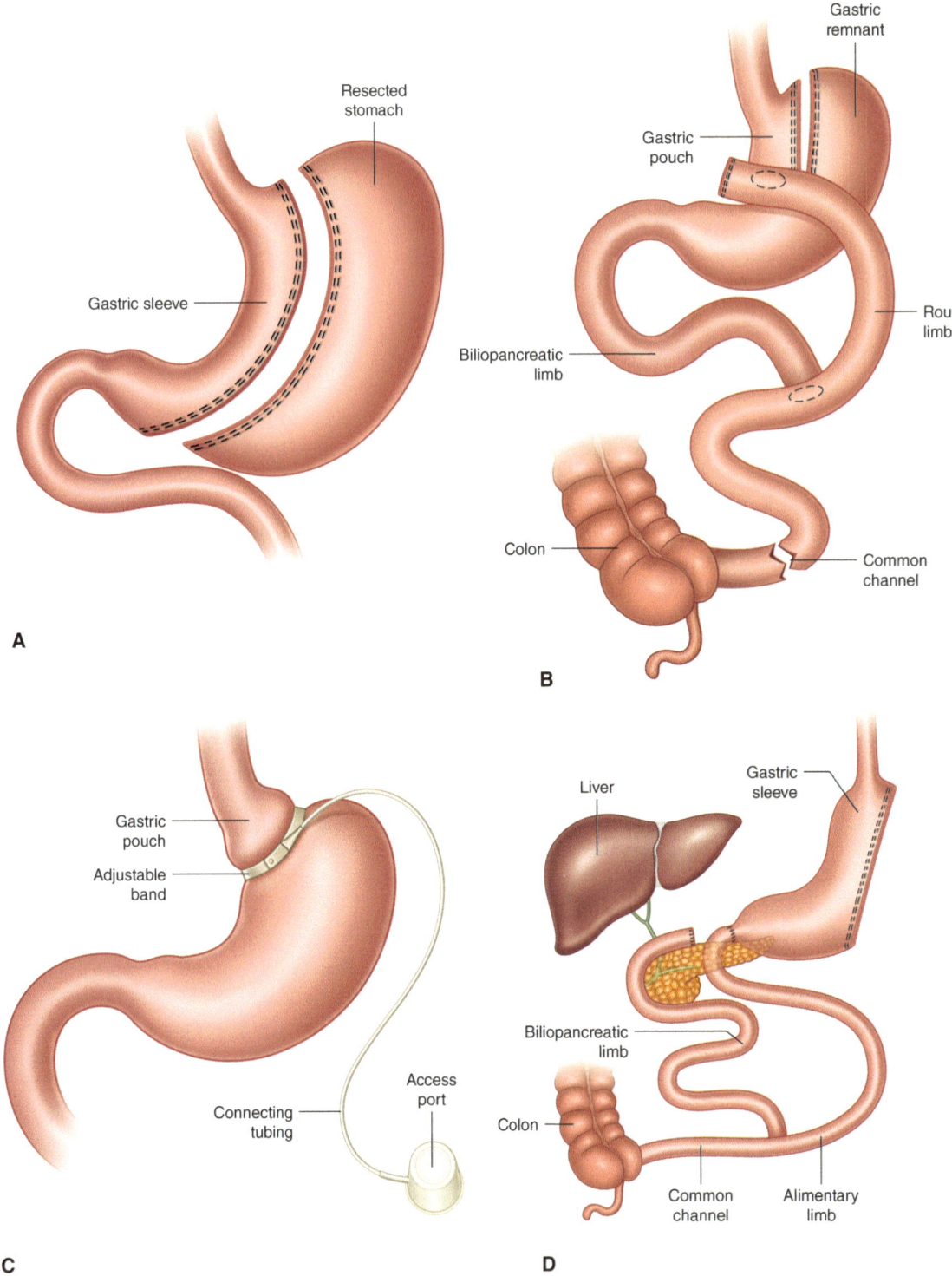

Fig. 5.1 Current bariatric operations. (**a**) Sleeve gastrectomy, (**b**) gastric bypass, (**c**) adjustable gastric band, (**d**) biliopancreatic diversion with duodenal switch

limited laparoscopic visualization, distortion of normal ana-tomical landmarks, and tissue friability. These difficult oper-ations should be converted to laparotomy, unless the surgeon has extensive prior experience in minimally invasive gastro-intestinal reconstruction.

Patient-related factors favoring laparotomy include hemodynamic instability, inability to tolerate pneumoperi-toneum, inadequate working space, the presence of signifi-cant adhesions, and inability to clearly identify anatomic structures.

Table 5.1 Operative complications of bariatric surgery

	Sleeve gastrectomy	Gastric bypass	Adjustable gastric band
Early complications (≤30 days)	Leak Sleeve obstruction (stricture or kink) Bleeding	Leak Bleeding Gastrojejunostomy stenosis Internal hernia Adhesions	Iatrogenic gastrointestinal perforation Dysphagia GERD
Late complications (>30 days)	GERD Stricture	Internal hernia Adhesions Marginal ulcer Gastrojejunostomy stenosis Trocar site hernia Intussusception	Band slippage (gastric prolapse) Esophageal or pouch dilation Band erosion Device malfunction GERD

GERD gastroesophageal reflux disease

Intraoperative decisions must account for anatomic changes due to weight loss, the location of the pathology, and the planned operation. The method of establishing pneumoperitoneum—open access, Veress needle technique, or direct optical entry—requires careful consideration. Weight loss depletes intra-abdominal adipose tissue leaving a redundant abdominal wall. Force applied to the abdominal wall during port placement can directly appose the surfaces of the abdominal wall and the retroperitoneum, allowing the possibility of injury to retroperitoneal structures. Consequently, open access for initial port placement is usually preferred. If Veress needle is used to create pneumoperitoneum, the risk of injuring retroperitoneal structures may be reduced by insertion in the left subcostal region along the midclavicular line. Once the pneumoperitoneum is established, the primary port is inserted using optical entry. Direct optical entry without insufflation is usually contraindicated.

The number and position of laparoscopic ports are determined by the planned operation and the intraoperative findings; however, unobstructed access to the common operative sites can be achieved using the port positions in Fig. 5.2. General guidelines for port placement are as follows: 5 and 12 mm right upper quadrant ports for the surgeon, two 5 mm left upper quadrant ports for the first assistant, a 12 mm supraumbilical port for the camera, and a 5 mm subxiphoid port for liver retraction. Initial exploration is completed using only the supraumbilical camera port and two right upper quadrant ports. If a laparoscopic approach appears feasible, the number and position of additional ports are determined by the patient's pathology. Often the subxiphoid port and/or the first assistant's port(s) can be eliminated. In addition, if inframesocolic pathology is suspected preoperatively, ports are shifted inferiorly 2–4 cm to provide better access to the inferior abdomen.

Gastrointestinal Leaks

Gastrointestinal leaks are a significant cause of morbidity and mortality following stapled bariatric operations. The location of the leak has both diagnostic and management implications. Leaks following sleeve gastrectomy most com-

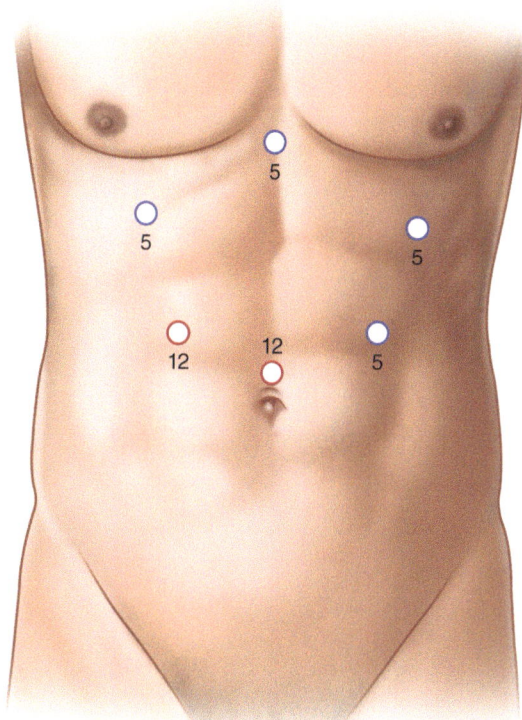

Fig. 5.2 Standard port positions for laparoscopic exploration following bariatric surgery

monly occur along the proximal staple line near the angle of His and are often associated with strictures at the gastric incisura. Leaks following gastric bypass most commonly occur at the gastrojejunostomy, but they can also occur at the jejunojejunostomy or any staple line.

Diagnosis

The presentation of gastrointestinal leak is a spectrum ranging from subtle clinical changes to septic shock. Early leaks can present with any combination of abdominal pain and tenderness, tachycardia, tachypnea, fever, and leukocytosis. Sinus tachycardia, defined as a sustained heart rate greater than 120 beats per minute, is the earliest and most sensitive finding. Late leaks can present more insidiously, often with only mild abdominal pain and fever.

Imaging is useful for both establishing the diagnosis and delineating the source of gastrointestinal leak. An upper gastrointestinal (UGI) series has limited utility in evaluating possible gastrointestinal leaks due to its poor sensitivity. Abdominal computed tomography (CT) is considered the best imaging modality for detecting gastrointestinal leaks (Fig. 5.3) [1]. However, interpretation of abdominal CT is influenced by the experience of the radiologist and by technical factors—including patient size and positioning, choice of oral/intravenous contrast, and timing of contrast

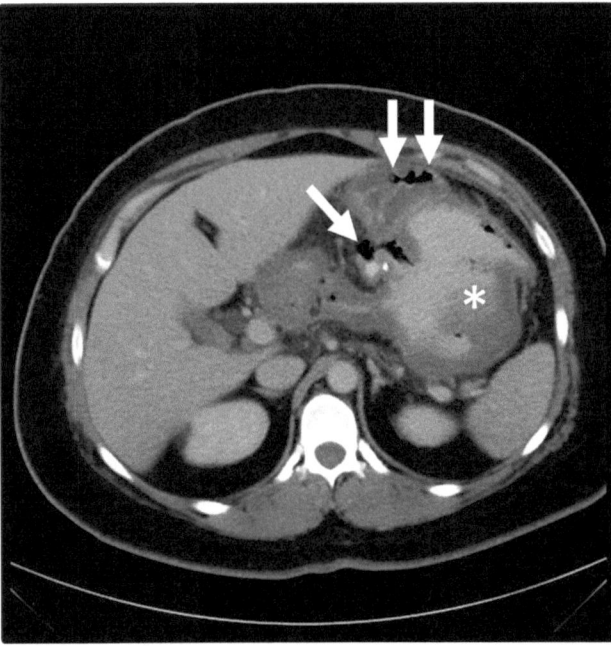

Fig. 5.3 Abdominal CT scan demonstrating a gastrojejunostomy leak following retrocolic, retrogastric gastric bypass. The axial view shows the gastric pouch (*single arrow*) is in direct continuity with the contrast-filled lesser sac collection (*). The gastric remnant (*double arrows*) is compressed by the lesser sac collection

administration. Despite these limitations, CT scan detection of sleeve gastrectomy leaks is excellent, with both high sensitivity and specificity. However, the results for detection of gastric bypass leaks are disappointing, missing up to one-third of leaks.

If imaging studies are unable to exclude gastrointestinal leaks or are not feasible due to the patient's habitus, operative exploration should be considered. The risks of a negative exploration are acceptable, given the consequences of delayed diagnosis.

Management of Gastrointestinal Leaks

Initial management of gastrointestinal leaks consists of bowel rest, fluid resuscitation, and broad-spectrum antimicrobial therapy. The acute management goals are to repair or control the gastrointestinal leak site, provide wide drainage, and establish access for nutritional support.

Non-operative management can be considered in patients with contained leaks who are hemodynamically normal and have no peritoneal findings. Acute non-operative treatment consists of bowel rest, broad-spectrum antimicrobial therapy, and nutritional support (either enteral or parenteral). Small intraperitoneal collections can be observed, but larger collections require percutaneous or operative drainage. Adjunctive endoscopic therapy can be used for the acute treatment of sleeve gastrectomy leaks (Fig. 5.4d) but is typically reserved for subacute or chronic leaks. Options include closure of the fistula tract using endoscopic suturing devices and clips and/or tissue sealant injection or exclusion of the fistula tract using covered endoscopic stents. Failure of non-operative management, heralded by increasing leukocytosis, increasing tachycardia, and worsening intra-abdominal pain or hemodynamic instability, is managed operatively.

Operative management of gastrointestinal leaks is influenced by the location of the leak and by the type of bariatric operation. Supramesocolic leaks encompass all sleeve leaks and any gastric bypass leak from the gastric pouch, gastrojejunostomy, or gastric remnant staple line. Inframesocolic leaks only occur following gastric bypass and originate from the jejunojejunostomy or the blind end of the biliopancreatic limb. Options for operative management of supramesocolic leaks include wide drainage alone, primary closure of the enteric defect with wide drainage, omental patching with wide drainage, or resection and primary anastomosis. The choice of operation depends on the patient's physiologic state and anatomic findings. Wide drainage alone (Fig. 5.4a) is reserved for patients that are clinically unstable or for those with inaccessible leak sites or a hostile abdomen. Primary repair is best suited for small, well-defined leaks but has a high failure rate due to friability of the tissue surrounding the leak site. Better alternatives are omental patching or

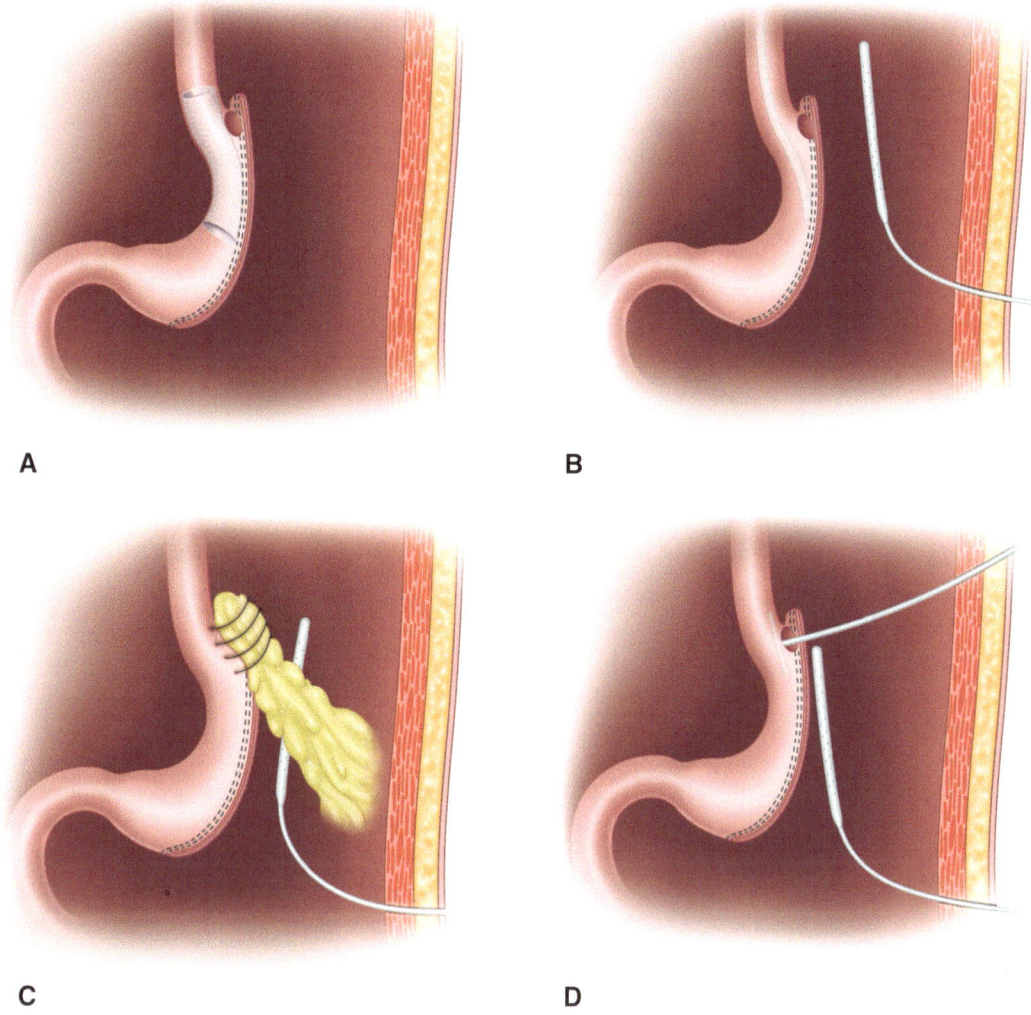

A

B

C

D

Fig. 5.4 Options for acute management of sleeve gastrectomy leaks. (**a**) Wide drainage without repair of leak site, (**b**) omental patch with wide drainage, (**c**) T-tube placement with wide drainage, (**d**) covered self-expanding endoscopic stent

placement of a T-tube to control the leak site in conjunction with wide drainage (Fig. 5.4b, c). Resection for the early management of supramesocolic leaks is rarely, if ever, necessary and should be avoided. The only exception is for gastric remnant staple line leaks, where resection through the normal gastric wall remote from the site of inflammation can be a definitive therapy.

Inframesocolic gastrointestinal leaks can be managed using any of the methods described above. However, the best option is usually resection with primary anastomosis. This operation has peculiarities related to the Roux limb anatomy. First, all mesentery must be preserved to avoid compromising the blood supply to the remaining Roux limb. Specifically, transection of the mesentery must be done as close to the bowel wall as possible. Second, reconstruction requires two bowel anastomoses: an anastomosis between the Roux limb and common channel and a second anastomosis between the biliopancreatic limb and common channel 20–30 cm distal to the first anastomosis. The location of biliopancreatic anastomosis is important. If the biliopancreatic anastomosis is placed proximal to the first anastomosis, the Roux limb is effectively shortened, which increases the risk of bile reflux.

Enteral access for nutritional support should be considered in all stable patients. Gastric remnant gastrostomy is possible in most gastric bypass patients. Tube jejunostomy is appropriate for sleeve gastrectomy patients and is an option for gastric bypass patients.

Postoperative Care

The postoperative care of the bariatric surgery patient with a gastrointestinal leak is similar to the management of gastrointestinal leaks in general surgery patients. Enteral feeding can be started as soon as the patient is hemodynamically normal. The duration of antibiotic therapy follows established institutional guidelines. Imaging studies can be used to evaluate whether leaks have sealed as well as to monitor resolution of any intra-abdominal collections. Alternatively, closure of the gastrointestinal leaks can be inferred, if the quality and quantity of drain output remain unchanged once a clear liquid diet is started. Drains are removed if the patient's clinical status remains stable after 1–2 days on oral intake. If the patient's gastrointestinal leak was controlled using a T-tube, the tube is withdrawn slowly when a well-defined fistula tract has formed, about 6 weeks after placement. Usually the fistula tract closes spontaneously, and, if not, fistula closure can be achieved using endoscopic techniques.

Gastrointestinal Obstruction

Gastrointestinal obstruction is a common complication after bariatric surgery. The differential diagnosis for obstruction is determined by the specific bariatric operation. The clinical presentation is influenced by both the specific etiology of the obstruction and the patient's bariatric operation. The clinical consequences of these potential etiologies determine the urgency of evaluation and management. The nuances of evaluation and management of obstruction are most easily understood when they are grouped according to the bariatric operation.

Obstruction After Gastric Bypass

The anatomy of the Roux-en-Y gastric bypass has significant implications for the evaluation and management of obstruction. Obstruction of the Roux limb or common channel produces typical obstructive symptoms and signs: nausea, vomiting, abdominal pain and tenderness, and distension [2]. Conversely, obstruction of the biliopancreatic limb produces vague early symptoms and signs: bloating, epigastric fullness, or pain. Later, typical obstructive symptoms may occur as the dilated gastric remnant distorts the proximal Roux limb creating a secondary obstruction.

Closed-loop obstructions are always a concern following gastric bypass. A Roux limb closed-loop obstruction may result when a complete obstruction occurs proximal to the jejunojejunostomy and the gastrojejunostomy is narrow. Complete obstruction of the biliopancreatic limb is always a closed-loop obstruction. Any patient with a suspected closed-loop obstruction, regardless of etiology, requires urgent intervention in order to minimize the risk of vascular compromise in the obstructed segment. Finally, any small bowel obstruction without an identifiable cause is assumed to be due to internal hernia and requires prompt abdominal exploration in order to avoid intestinal strangulation.

The loss of working space, resulting from obstruction and subsequent dilation of the Roux limb, biliopancreatic limb, and/or gastric remnant, is an intraoperative challenge regardless of the etiology of obstruction. Laparotomy may be required, unless these dilated regions can be decompressed. The Roux limb can sometimes be decompressed using a nasogastric tube passed across the gastrojejunostomy under laparoscopic guidance. An alternative is laparoscopic aspiration of the Roux limb using a gallbladder aspiration needle to puncture the bowel along its anti-mesenteric boarder. Once the limb is decompressed, the needle puncture site is repaired with a figure-of-eight suture. The gastric remnant and biliopancreatic limb can be decompressed using a remnant gastrostomy tube.

Gastrojejunal Anastomotic Stricture

Gastrojejunal anastomotic strictures are a common complication after gastric bypass, occurring in up to 15% of patients, usually within 3 months of surgery. Patients describe solid food intolerance that progresses to liquid intolerance as the stricture worsens over time.

Upper endoscopy is the preferred method for diagnosis and treatment. Following endoscopic confirmation of stricture, the gastrojejunostomy is sequentially dilated with through-the-scope hydrostatic balloon dilators, with the goal of achieving a 12–15 mm dilation. Stricture dilation requires sufficient anastomotic scar disruption to prevent recurrent stricture while avoiding anastomotic perforation. Practically, a dilation session should be terminated once the dilation goal has been achieved or when anastomotic bleeding, indicating the limit of safe dilation, is seen when the balloon is deflated.

Patients receiving endoscopic dilation are started on a full liquid diet in the recovery room and are advanced as tolerated. If oral intake is adequate, further treatments can be completed on an outpatient basis. Most patients need only a single treatment session to prevent recurrent stricture; a smaller percentage will require multiple dilation sessions at 2-week intervals. Only about 5% of patients will need surgical revision. Any patient reporting significant abdominal pain immediately following dilation warrants an imaging study to exclude the possibility of inadvertent perforation.

Internal Hernia

Internal hernia occurs when the small intestine passes through mesenteric spaces formed during creation of a Roux-en-Y gastric bypass (Fig. 5.5). The number of potential hernia sites is determined by the position of the Roux limb, with respect to the transverse colon: two potential defects exist for an antecolic Roux limb, and there are three for a retrocolic

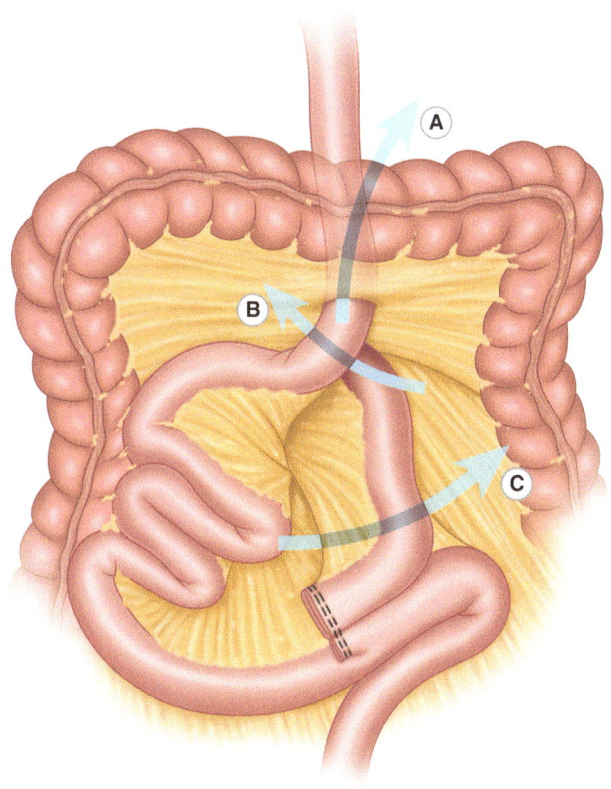

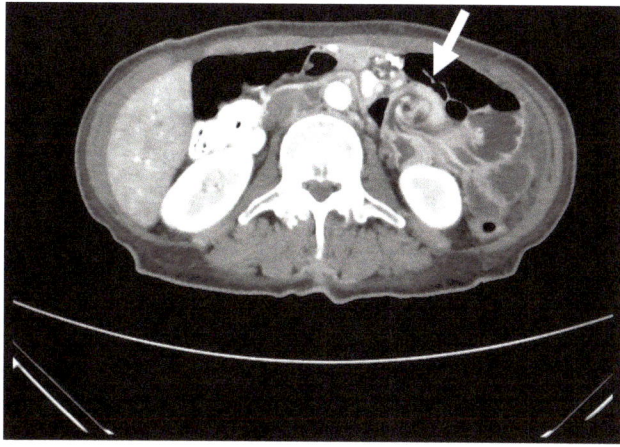

Fig. 5.6 Abdominal CT demonstrating mesenteric vascular spiraling (*arrow*)—"swirl sign"—suggestive of internal hernia

Fig. 5.5 Potential sites for internal hernia following gastric bypass. (**a**) Transverse mesocolic defect, (**b**) Petersen's space, (**c**) jejunojejunostomy mesenteric defect

Roux limb. Both antecolic and retrocolic gastric bypasses have potential defects in the small bowel mesentery at the jejunojejunostomy and at Petersen's space—a triangular opening bounded by the Roux limb mesentery, transverse mesocolon, and retroperitoneum. Retrocolic gastric bypass has an additional potential space created by passage of the Roux limb through the transverse mesocolon.

Internal hernias are the most common cause of small bowel obstruction following gastric bypass. They occur more commonly following laparoscopic gastric bypass, compared with open gastric bypass. The peak incidence for presentation occurs between 6 and 24 months postoperatively.

The diagnosis of internal hernia can be difficult, due to its highly variable acute and chronic symptoms. Patients can present acutely with the sudden onset of severe abdominal pain, sometimes associated with obstructive symptoms. They can also present with chronic abdominal pain alone. Physical examination reveals focal periumbilical or epigastric tenderness. Significant abdominal distension is usually absent, even with obstructive symptoms, due to the proximal location of the obstruction. Laboratory studies are not usually helpful. Leukocytosis or lactic acidosis suggests ischemia of the entrapped intestine.

Abdominal CT has replaced upper gastrointestinal series as the preferred imaging study. Findings of internal hernia include (1) displacement of the jejunojejunostomy staple lines into the right abdomen, (2) clustered loops of the small intestine in the left upper quadrant, (3) small bowel loops posterior to the superior mesenteric artery, and (4) mesenteric vascular spiraling known as the "swirl sign" (Fig. 5.6). However, reliance on imaging studies should be cautioned, since up to 20% of patients with internal hernia will have imaging studies interpreted as normal. Accordingly, urgent abdominal exploration remains the definitive diagnostic tool for gastric bypass patients with suspected internal hernia [3]. The consequences of intestinal strangulation from delayed diagnosis far outweigh the risks associated with a negative abdominal exploration.

Prior to surgery, nearly all patients require fluid and electrolyte repletion, due to poor oral intake. The use of nasogastric tubes is relatively contraindicated, due to the risk of placement-related perforation of the pouch or Roux limb. However, if the patient has obstruction and has a significant aspiration risk, nasogastric decompression can be accomplished using fluoroscopic guidance.

The laparoscopic management of suspected internal hernia proceeds in four steps: (1) determine the position of the Roux limb, (2) reduce the internal hernia, (3) assess intestinal viability, and (4) eliminate all potential sites for recurrent hernia. On initial exploration, it is essential to establish whether the Roux limb is in an antecolic or retrocolic position. This dictates the number of potential sites of internal hernia that need to be addressed later in the procedure. The next step is to reduce the internal hernia. While it is tempting to attack the internal hernia directly, the urge should be avoided. Distortion of the anatomy makes accurate identification of the involved structures difficult. A more reliable method to safely reduce the hernia is to identify the ileocecal valve and then run the bowel proximally along the common channel. During this process, the internal hernia will be reduced. Upon completion of the maneuver, the intestine will be in its normal anatomic position. Occasionally, the maneuver cannot be completed, due to bowel wall edema or adhesions, and laparotomy will be necessary. The third step is to assess the intestinal viability. If a nonviable bowel is present, prompt conversion to laparotomy for further assessment and possible resection is indicated. Finally, all potential sites of internal hernia are closed with permanent suture. Mesentery should be coapted without significant tension, using either running or interrupted suture. Closing the space between the Roux limb and gastric remnant is not necessary. Finally, it is desirable to avoid gaps in the suture lines when closing the mesenteric defects. These gaps can enlarge to create new potential hernia sites as a result of mesenteric adipose tissue depletion during subsequent weight loss.

Internal hernia occurring through defects that had been closed during prior operations (i.e., recurrent internal hernia or primary internal hernia in patients who had the Petersen's space and the mesenteric defects closed during the original operation) is a vexing challenge. One approach to this challenge is a repair of the hernia defect using two layers of permanent suture. An alternative approach is the application of fibrin glue as an adjunct to a one-layer closure. Unfortunately, there is little existing data to support the effectiveness of either approach.

Patients managed using a laparoscopic approach can resume oral intake within 24 h of surgery and can be discharged within 1–2 days. If a decompressive gastrostomy tube was placed, it is capped once the output is negligible, and the tube can be removed 6 weeks postoperatively. Recurrent hernias can occur despite adequate mesenteric closure and must be considered if patients become symptomatic in the future.

Adhesions

Adhesions are the second most common cause of small bowel obstruction after gastric bypass. The site of obstruction affects the clinical presentation, as described above. Abdominal CT scan may be useful in localizing the transition zone. Patients with closed-loop obstructions or uncertain diagnosis require urgent operative therapy. In addition, operative therapy should be considered for all early small bowel obstructions to avoid anastomotic or staple line blowout.

Uncommon Causes of Small Bowel Obstruction

Intussusception is an uncommon cause of small bowel obstruction after gastric bypass. Both antegrade intussusception of the Roux limb and retrograde intussusception of the common channel into the jejunojejunostomy have been described. In most cases, there is no pathologic abnormality of the lead point. A "target sign" (Fig. 5.7) on abdominal CT scan is pathognomonic. Optimal operative therapy has not been established. Both resection and small bowel plication have been described. A reasonable approach for retrograde intussusceptions is plication of the common channel to the biliopancreatic limb for about 20 cm distal to the jejunojejunostomy.

Intraluminal hematoma obstructing the jejunojejunostomy is a rare cause of early postoperative small bowel obstruction. Abdominal CT with oral contrast (Fig. 5.8) will show a non-enhancing intraluminal mass with dilation of the Roux limb and/or the biliopancreatic limb. The obstruction is relieved by evacuating the hematoma through a nearby enterotomy or by reopening the jejunojejunostomy.

Obstruction After Sleeve Gastrectomy

Common causes of obstruction after sleeve gastrectomy are stricture—typically near the gastric incisura—and kinking of the sleeve. While nausea and vomiting are common following sleeve gastrectomy, the diagnosis should be suspected in patients with intractable symptoms. Diagnosis is confirmed by upper gastrointestinal series. Initial management is bowel rest and intravenous hydration. Occasionally, fluoroscopically placed nasogastric decompression is needed. Definitive management of this challenging problem

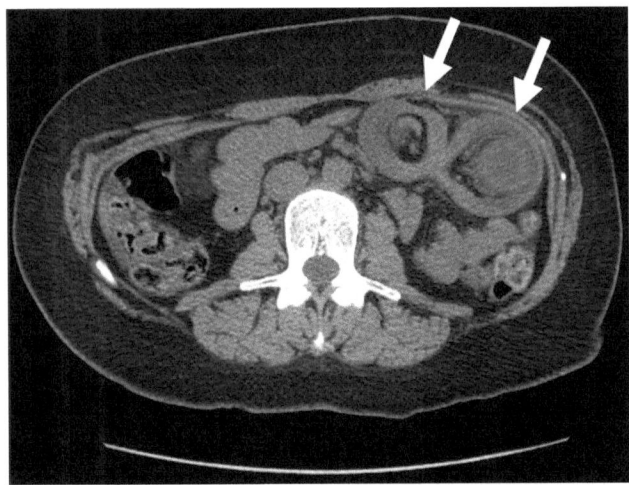

Fig. 5.7 Abdominal CT scan with "target signs" (*arrows*) indicative of jejunal intussusception

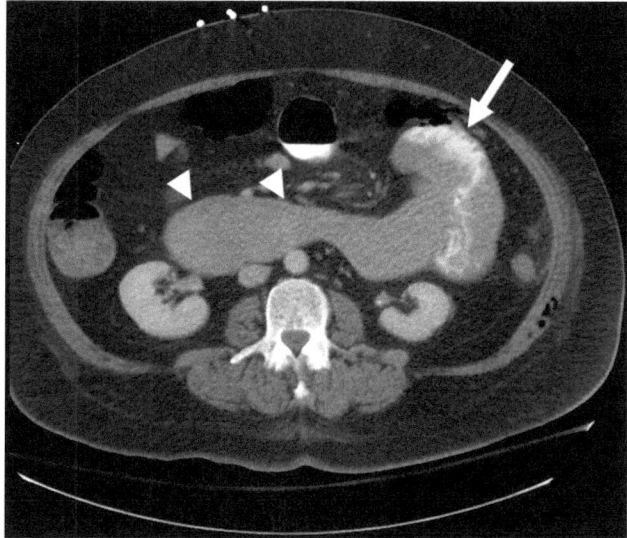

Fig. 5.8 Abdominal CT scan showing intraluminal hematoma. Contrast (*arrow*) outlines the intraluminal hematoma occupying the jejunojejunostomy. The duodenum (*arrowheads*) and gastric remnant (not shown) are dilated, diagnostic of a closed-loop obstruction

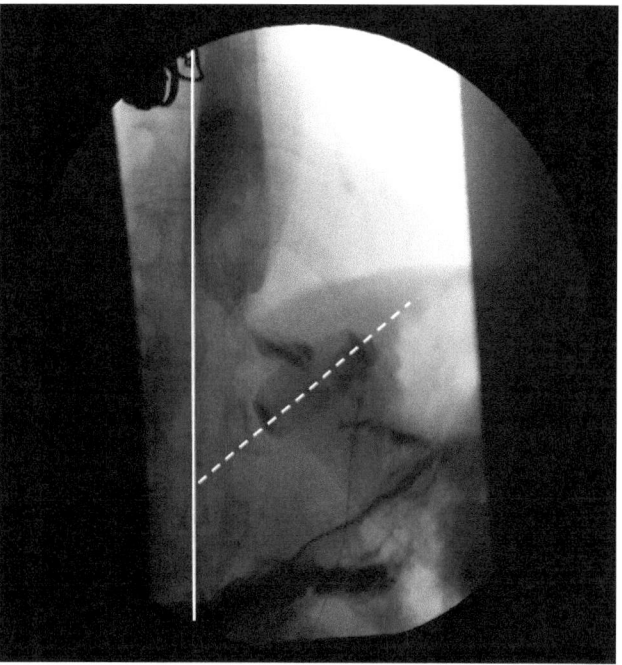

Fig. 5.9 Fluoroscopic image during UGI series demonstrating normal adjustable gastric band position. *Solid lines* indicate the horizontal and vertical axes. The axis of the gastric band, seen in profile overlying the contrast-filled proximal stomach, is 45° from vertical, directed toward the left shoulder (*dashed line*)

requires significant experience and should prompt referral to a bariatric surgeon. Strictures have been successfully managed with a combination of endoscopic dilation and stent placement. Kinks have been successfully managed using laparoscopic adhesiolysis with concurrent endoscopic stent placement. Conversion to gastric bypass is the definitive therapy for treatment failures.

Obstruction After Adjustable Gastric Banding

Obstruction after adjustable gastric banding is due to band slippage (gastric prolapse) or overfilling the band. Patients present with intractable nausea and vomiting. Alteration of the band position on abdominal radiograph suggests band slippage. On plain abdominal film, the normal band is seen in profile with the long axis directed toward the left shoulder and angled about 45 degrees from vertical (Fig. 5.9). A vertically positioned band suggests a posterior gastric prolapse, while a horizontally positioned band suggests anterior gastric prolapse. UGI series confirms the diagnosis, showing an enlarged asymmetrical pouch. Patients with an overfilled band have a normal band position on plain abdominal film. UGI series demonstrates symmetrical dilation of the gastric pouch and, sometimes, the esophagus. However, extensive radiologic evaluation is generally unnecessary since complete deflation of the band at the bedside will eliminate symptoms in most patients. Subsequently, a bariatric surgeon can electively correct the underlying source of obstruction by band removal, band revision, or conversion to a stapled bariatric operation.

Marginal Ulceration

Introduction

Marginal ulcer following gastric bypass occurs at the gastrojejunostomy, typically on the jejunal side of the anastomosis. The reported incidence of marginal ulceration is between 0.5 and 16%. This probably underestimates the true incidence of the complication, as up to 30% of patients are asymptomatic. Most marginal ulcers present within the first year following gastric bypass; few occur after the first year. Common risk factors are the use of tobacco or nonsteroidal anti-inflammatory drugs. Suspected risk factors include an excessively large gastric pouch, H. pylori infection, alcohol use, steroids, and possibly anticoagulation.

Diagnosis

Uncomplicated marginal ulcer typically presents with epigastric abdominal pain and tenderness, often associated with nausea and vomiting. Laboratory findings are typically unremarkable, though mild chronic anemia may result from chronic blood loss. Patients with mild typical symptoms can be given a trial of empiric treatment. However, upper endoscopy is appropriate for most patients, both to confirm the diagnosis and to establish a

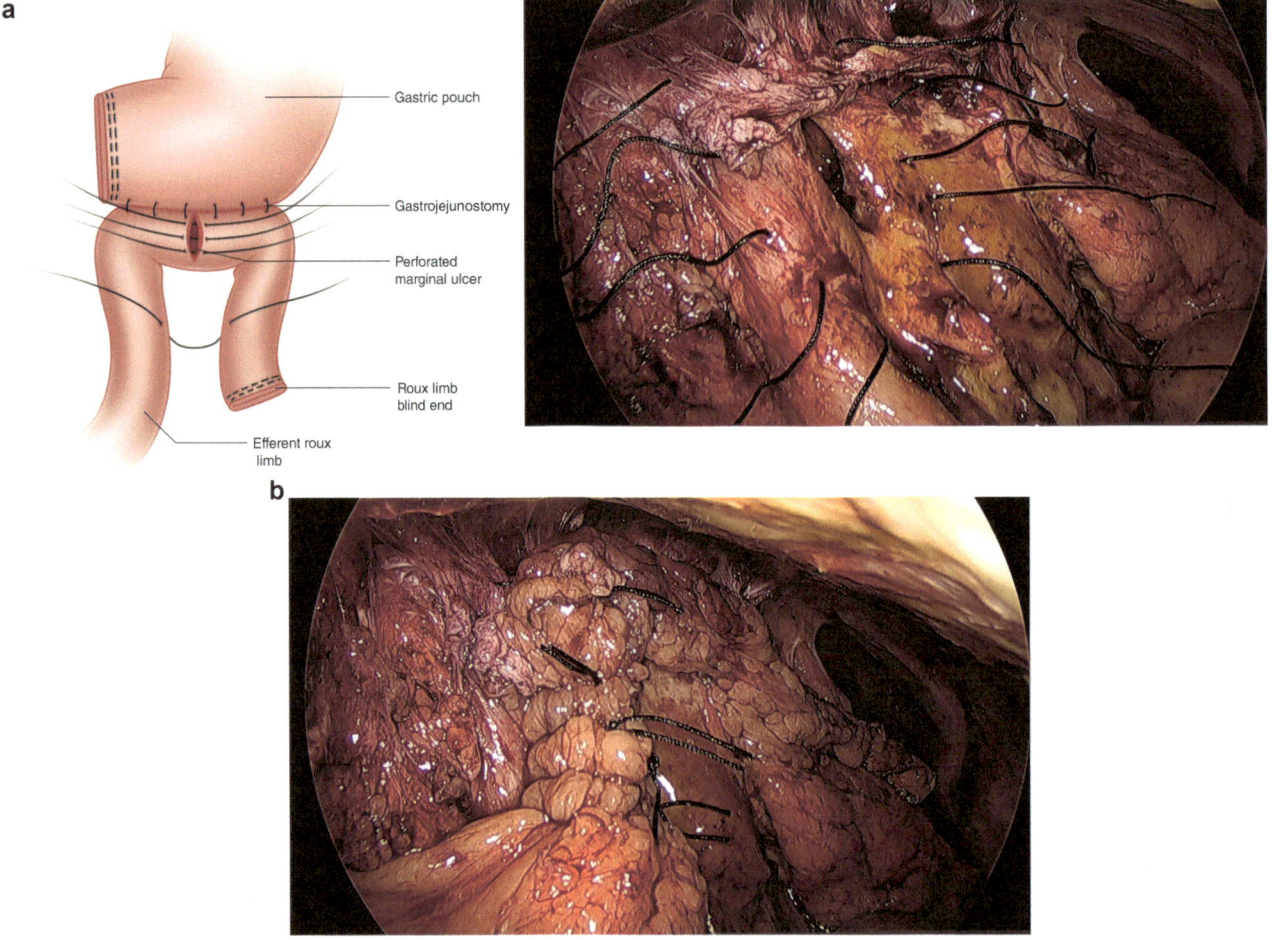

Fig. 5.10 Treatment of a perforated marginal ulcer with an omental patch. (**a**) The 2 cm perforation located just distal to the gastrojejunostomy with pre-placed sutures. (**b**) The sutures are tied over the omental pedicle to complete the repair

baseline to assess therapeutic response. Complications of marginal ulcer include perforation, bleeding, or intractability.

Patients with perforation often give an antecedent history consistent with marginal ulcer, followed by a sudden onset of generalized abdominal pain. Physical examination varies from moderate local tenderness to generalized peritonitis. Upright chest X-ray or abdominal plain films usually demonstrate free air. Further imaging is not normally indicated; however, in atypical cases, CT scan with oral contrast may show inflammation at the gastrojejunostomy with free air, peritoneal fluid, and contrast leak.

Bleeding ulcers present similarly to duodenal ulcers. Upper endoscopy is used to confirm the diagnosis and as a therapeutic intervention. The role for tagged red blood cell scans or angiography is limited.

Management

Most uncomplicated marginal ulcers respond to medical therapy, typically a combination of a proton pump inhibitor (PPI) and sucralfate. Ulcers normally heal within 12 weeks. Those that fail initial therapy often respond to a higher dose or a different PPI. Elective resection is reserved for intractable ulcers.

Bleeding ulcers often stop bleeding spontaneously. Those that continue to bleed actively respond to endoscopic therapy using epinephrine injection or endoscopic clips. Once bleeding is controlled, management is identical to that for uncomplicated marginal ulcers. Uncontrolled or recurrent bleeding is managed with urgent or emergent resection.

Options for treatment of perforated marginal ulcers include primary repair, with or without omental buttress, omental patching, or resection. Primary repair of small perforations using absorbable or permanent suture, buttressed with the pedicle of omentum, has been reported. More often, the perforation is too large, or the inflammation is too intense to allow primary repair. In these cases, the defect can be patched with an omental pedicle (Fig. 5.10) created to allow tension-free coverage of the defect [4]. The omental pedicle is secured using a row of interrupted, full-thickness permanent or absorbable sutures that straddle the perforation. All sutures can be placed prior to position the omental pedicle, or, alternatively, they can be placed and tied sequentially. The former allows more precise suture placement at the risk of entangling the sutures. Ulcers that are too large or are too friable for omental patch repair are candidates for resection of the ulcer. This involves resecting the distal pouch, gastrojejunostomy, and proximal Roux limb. The use of drains following repair is not well studied, so drains should be used at the surgeon's discretion. A reasonable approach is to drain only patients with high-risk closures (e.g., those involving highly friable tissue) or those with severe peritoneal contamination.

Postoperative Care

Patients having surgery for bleeding or perforated marginal ulcers may be started on a clear liquid diet 1–2 days following surgery. The quality and quantity of drain output are monitored, and, if unchanged, drains are removed prior to discharge. Follow-up imaging studies are not usually necessary. The duration of antibiotic therapy follows the established institutional guidelines.

Lifelong proton pump inhibitors should be considered for all patients with complicated marginal ulcer. Testing for *H. pylori* prior to discharge is a routine, and standard treatment is started for affected patients. Risk factor modification, especially the elimination of tobacco and nonsteroidal anti-inflammatory drug use, is essential to minimize the risk of recurrent marginal ulcer.

Take-Home Messages

1. Gastrointestinal leaks following bariatric surgery have a highly variable clinical presentation, from minimal abdominal complaints to generalized peritonitis. Because imaging studies often miss small leaks, abdominal exploration is a standard diagnostic tool. The risks of a negative exploration are acceptable, given the disastrous consequences of delayed diagnosis.
2. Internal hernia is the cause of any small bowel obstruction following laparoscopic gastric bypass until excluded. Often this requires surgical exploration, because imaging studies commonly miss the diagnosis. The risks of a negative exploration are acceptable given the risk of intestinal strangulation due to delayed diagnosis.
3. Band deflation is often the only acute intervention needed for obstructive symptoms following adjustable gastric banding. Definitive management is performed electively.
4. Avoid tunnel vision! Not all acute intra-abdominal processes are related to a bariatric operation. Look for other things.

Key References

1. Kim J, Azagury D, Eisenberg D, DeMaria E, Campos GM. ASMBS position statement on prevention, detection, and treatment of gastrointestinal leak after gastric bypass and sleeve gastrectomy, including the roles of imaging, surgical exploration, and nonoperative management. Surg Obes Relat Dis. 2015;11:739–48.
2. Agaba EA, Gentles CV, Shamseddeen H, Sasthakonar V, Kandel A, Gadelata D, Gellman L. Retrospective analysis of abdominal pain in postoperative laparoscopic Roux-en-Y gastric bypass patients: is a simple algorithm the answer? Surg Obes Relat Dis. 2008;4:587–93.
3. Gandhi AD, Patel RA, Brolin RE. Elective laparoscopy for herald symptoms of mesenteric/internal hernia after laparoscopic Roux-en-Y gastric bypass. Surg Obes Relat Dis. 2009;5:144–9.
4. Moon RC, Teixeira AF, Goldbach M, Jawad MA. Management and treatment outcomes of marginal ulcers after Roux-en-Y gastric bypass at a single high volume bariatric center. Surg Obes Relat Dis. 2014;10:229–34.

Chad G. Ball, Francis R. Sutherland, and S. Morad Hameed

Introduction

Minimally invasive, or laparoscopic, cholecystectomy is currently the most frequent general surgical operation performed within the abdomen. It is also the most common intraperitoneal operation performed by our surgical trainees. Despite this reality, inflammation of the gallbladder and surrounding structures can make this seemingly straightforward operation both daunting and dangerous.

It is estimated that only 1–4% of asymptomatic or mildly symptomatic patients will develop an acute complication of cholelithiasis. This may include acute cholecystitis (AC), cholangitis, and/or pancreatitis (with AC being the most frequent). It is interesting to note that a recent population-based study showed a global decline in the incidence of all severe cholelithiasis-related complications. This was primarily based on a reduction in AC due to the widespread adoption of laparoscopic cholecystectomy. Conversely, the incidence of acute biliary pancreatitis and cholangitis has increased during the same interval.

Acute inflammation of the gallbladder is a frequent complication of cholelithiasis and affects up to 20% of patients with recurrent symptomatic gallstones. Despite the history that most patients provide (previous episodes of transient colic pain in their right upper quadrant), acute presentations to a healthcare facility are typically longer and associated with additional symptoms (nausea or vomiting after ingesting high-fat foods). Obstruction of the cystic duct by a gallstone or sludge produces dilation of the gallbladder and increases its internal pressure. Subsequent biliary stasis and the proliferation of microorganisms are typical. If the obstruction persists, venous outflow decreases, with dilatation of capillaries and lymphatics resulting in gallbladder wall edema and thickening. Eventually the gallbladder develops areas of hemorrhage and necrosis due to vascular occlusion. Imaging and exploration may reveal both fluid and air within the gallbladder wall. If the ischemia and necrosis are located within the posterior wall (i.e., apposed to the liver), a pericholecystic abscess eroding into the liver can occur. It is also important to note that specific complications such as perforation, biliary peritonitis, pericholecystic abscess, and biliary fistula (between the gallbladder and duodenum, colon, and stomach) may alter the clinical presentation and increase morbidity and mortality of the disease. Bouveret's syndrome, gastric outlet obstruction, biliary ileus, and gallstone-related small bowel obstruction are uncommon complications.

Preoperative Diagnostic Options

Similar to trauma, the initial evaluation of patients presenting with a gallbladder emergency should include simultaneous diagnosis and therapy. This concurrent rapid assessment and treatment are particularly important for patients who present with profound sepsis (gangrenous cholecystitis or cholangitis). A detailed clinical history of the acute event, including a focused past medical history (i.e., history of gallstones, pancreatitis, duodenal ulcer/NSAID use, and/or cancer), and complete physical examination are crucial. These details may suggest the likely diagnosis, determine the severity of the acute event, and guide both immediate and subsequent treatments. It is important to note that most patients present with an inflammatory and/or septic complication of a previously known disease, as opposed to a completely de novo etiology. Thus, patients presenting with AC or another complication of gallstones typically have a known history of symptomatic cholelithiasis. By contrast, patients suffering from pancreatic diseases generally develop symptoms after an acute new event.

C.G. Ball (✉) • F.R. Sutherland
Foothills Medical Center, Department of Surgery,
Calgary, AB, Canada
e-mail: ball.chad@gmail.com

S. Morad Hameed
Vancouver General Hospital, Department of Trauma,
Vancouver, BC, Canada

K.A. Khwaja, J.J. Diaz (eds.), *Minimally Invasive Acute Care Surgery*, https://doi.org/10.1007/978-3-319-64723-4_6

The first step in caring for these patients requires a direct assessment of the severity of the acute event itself. Septic shock represents the most common causes of hemodynamic compromise and must be addressed immediately. These methodologies include intravenous fluid resuscitation, early initiation of antimicrobial therapy, and blood product transfusion as needed. It is important to highlight that these patients often present with nausea and vomiting, dehydration, acute kidney injury, electrolyte imbalances, anemia, and/or coagulation abnormalities.

Once effectively resuscitated, patients should undergo diagnostic imaging tests to rapidly determine the precise etiology and guide further treatment. This initial diagnostic assessment includes two dominant objectives: (1) confirming the diagnosis and (2) establishing its severity. Despite a wide array of options (US, HIDA, CT, MR), the revised Tokyo consensus guidelines represent the best parameters for directing diagnosis and treatment. Based on diagnostic sensitivities of 90–95%, abdominal US remains the initial modality of choice. Because US can be performed by the acute care surgeon within the emergency department, it is also cost saving and rapid. Identification of gallbladder wall thickening (> 5 mm), an obstructing gallstone in the gallbladder neck, pericholecystic fluid, US Murphy's sign, and/or dilation and thickening of the common bile duct (CBD) are important signs that contribute to defining the diagnosis of AC. Unfortunately, CT imaging is far less specific and helpful. Furthermore, HIDA is rarely needed but can be of occasional assistance in cases of nondiagnostic US in the context of a high pretest probability for AC. Findings of complete non-filling of the gallbladder are diagnostic for complete occlusion of the cystic duct and therefore AC. After confirmation, however, AC should be classified according its severity (grade I, mild; II, moderate; III, severe). While grade II refers to the presence of systemic signs of inflammation, grade III cholecystitis includes dysfunction of at least one organ/system (Table 6.1).

The presence of *jaundice* concurrent to AC should be evaluated with caution because it reflects a wide spectrum of potentially benign and malignant conditions. These include, but are not limited to, CBD obstruction from external compression (cholangiocarcinoma, periampullary cancers, gallbladder cancer), choledocholithiasis, and liver failure (e.g., secondary to sepsis). Although US continues to be the diagnostic gold standard for detecting choledocholithiasis, MR cholangiography (MRC) may also be useful to define the etiology. The dominant goals in the treatment of patients with choledocholithiasis are threefold: (1) treat concurrent sepsis, (2) evacuate the CBD, and (3) prevent future recurrences. Although the order of the latter two goals is debated on the basis of length of stay, safety, and economics, it is clear that ERCP and laparoscopic cholecystectomy represent the two dominant therapies. Laparoscopic CBD exploration

Table 6.1 Severity assessment criteria for acute cholecystitis

Grade	Definition
I (mild)	Acute cholecystitis does not meet the criteria of "grade III" or "grade II" It can also be defined as acute cholecystitis in a healthy patient with no organ dysfunction and mild inflammatory changes in the gallbladder, making cholecystectomy a safe and low-risk operative procedure
II (moderate)	Acute cholecystitis is associated with any one of the following conditions: 1. Elevated white blood cell count (>18,000/mm³) 2. Palpable tender mass in the right upper abdominal quadrant 3. Duration of complaints >72 h 4. Marked local inflammation (gangrenous cholecystitis, pericholecystic abscess, hepatic abscess, biliary peritonitis, emphysematous cholecystitis)
III (severe)	"Grade III" (severe) acute cholecystitis is associated with dysfunction of any one of the following organs/systems 1. Cardiovascular dysfunction defined as hypotension requiring treatment with dopamine ≥5 µg/kg per min or any dose of norepinephrine 2. Neurological dysfunction defined as decreased level of consciousness 3. Respiratory dysfunction defined as a PaO_2/FiO_2 ratio < 300 4. Renal dysfunction defined as oliguria, creatinine >2.0 mg/dl 5. Hepatic dysfunction defined as PT-INR > 1.5 6. Hematological dysfunction defined as platelet count <100,000/mm³

(transcystic or transductal) is also a viable option and has the added benefit of being performed as a single procedure.

Acalculous cholecystitis is an uncommon and serious presentation observed in 5–10% of patients with biliary emergencies. It is typically associated with critical illness, immunosuppressive conditions, uncommon pathogens (anaerobes), and/or sepsis. On a global basis, patients with acquired immunodeficiency syndrome (AIDS) continue to represent the most common immunosuppressive cases and are younger, present with elevations in their alkaline phosphatase and serum bilirubin, and may have cytomegalovirus- and cryptosporidium-associated infections. Other rare causes of acalculous cholecystitis are chemical cholecystitis after hepatic artery infusion, antibiotic-related cholecystitis, and parasites (*Ascaris*). Since patients with acalculous cholecystitis often present with organ dysfunction and are poor surgical candidates, medical treatment is often the therapy of choice, with surgery performed in selected cases (i.e., if cholecystostomy is ineffective).

Pregnant patients carry a higher risk of developing both gallstones and AC than nonpregnant patients. Complications of gallstones remain the second most common cause of surgery during pregnancy. Despite this epidemiology, surgery should be avoided during the first (may result in abortion) and third (may result in premature delivery) trimesters if possible. Most symptomatic patients treated with nonoperative therapy present with recurrence of their symptoms however. Of this cohort, approximately 30% eventually require surgery during their pregnancy.

Management

The treatment of patients with AC should include general medical therapy (nil per mouth (NPO), intravenous fluids, antibiotics, and analgesia) followed by urgent cholecystectomy. The two dominant surgical issues include the type (open vs. laparoscopic) and timing (early vs. delayed) of the procedure. Two small prospective randomized trials compared open with laparoscopic surgery for AC. The first study showed that open cholecystectomy had a significantly higher number of postoperative complications, as well as a longer postoperative hospital stay (6 vs. 4 days). No mortality or bile duct injuries were observed. A more recent trial included 70 patients and did not show any significant difference in the rate of postoperative complications. The laparoscopic group had a significantly longer median operating time (90 vs. 80 min) and shorter median postoperative stay. The timing of cholecystectomy has also been evaluated in prospective randomized trials. Numerous small studies have observed that patients undergoing early cholecystectomy have a shorter hospital stay, without any other significant differences. A recent meta-analysis that included 451 patients from five trials comparing early (less than 7 days from the onset of symptoms) with delayed (more than 6 weeks after the index admission) cholecystectomy revealed no statistically significant difference between the groups with regard to bile duct injuries (BDIs) or conversion to open surgery. The hospital stay was 3 days shorter in the early group however. Importantly, 40 (17.5%) patients in the delayed group required an emergency cholecystectomy during their waiting period for non-resolving or recurrent AC. It is also evident from large population-based studies that the rate of BDI increases with higher grades of cholecystitis. The most recent prospective multicenter trial comparing the optimal timing for cholecystectomy (early, during the first 24 h vs. delayed) in patients with AC confirmed that early cholecystectomy was associated with significantly lower morbidity (11.8 vs. 34.4%). Furthermore, while the conversion to open surgery and mortality rates were similar between groups, the mean length of hospital stay (5.4 vs. 10 days) and hospital costs were also significantly lower in the group treated with early cholecystectomy. In summary, although 30-day postoperative morbidity and mortality may remain independent of timing, it is clear that patients who undergo laparoscopic cholecystectomy beyond 24 h of acute inflammation are more likely to require an open procedure and sustain significantly longer postoperative and overall lengths of hospital admission and therefore cost. Taken together, these results suggest that early laparoscopic surgery should be considered the treatment of choice for acute care surgeons (ACS).

The role of antibiotic prophylaxis prior to elective laparoscopic cholecystectomy has been studied in prospective randomized trials. Unfortunately, the evidence remains insufficient to either support or refute their use in an attempt to reduce surgical site and global infections. This question has not been evaluated for patients undergoing urgent cholecystectomy for AC in any trials however. As a result, consensus guidelines recommend that antibiotic therapy should be started if infection is suspected on the basis of clinical, laboratory, and/or radiographic findings. Treatment should include coverage for the *Enterobacteriaceae* family (i.e., second-generation cephalosporin or a combination of a quinolone and metronidazole). Prophylaxis for enterococci is debated. Elderly patients and those with diabetes mellitus or immunosuppressive disorders should receive antibiotics even when infection has not been confirmed. Obtaining aerobic and anaerobic cultures from the bile during surgery is also recommended to guide complex cases.

In summary, patients with grade I or II AC should undergo early laparoscopic cholecystectomy, with awareness of the extent of the gallbladder's inflammation. More specifically, the ACS surgeon must be particularly wary of the inflamed gallbladder that is contracted into the liver bed upon initial laparoscopic inspections because the anatomy in this scenario represents the most common etiology for BDI. Patients with grade III AC should undergo cholecystectomy once organ dysfunction is reversed. In the setting of persistent organ failure or poor surgical candidacy, antimicrobial therapy and concurrent ultrasound-guided percutaneous cholecystostomy should be performed.

The technical elements of performing a laparoscopic cholecystectomy are cemented in both lessons learned from BDI and from preceptor-based preferences. While port/trocar placement varies widely between surgeons, the most common locations for a four-port technique are the epigastrium (5 mm), right flank (5 mm), supraumbilical (5, 10 or 12 mm), and midway between the xiphoid process and umbilicus at a location to the right of the midline (5 mm). As the patients become more obese, this final port is generally moved more laterally to improve triangulation for a gallbladder located within a fatty liver. The issue of visual alignment and perspective has become even more topical with the proliferation of single-incision laparoscopic cholecystectomy which is known to be associated with a higher rate of common bile duct injury than a traditional four-incision laparoscopic technique utilizing an angled scope.

Injury avoidance is clearly the stated goal of every ACS surgeon embarking upon an urgent cholecystectomy. While much has been written about preventing BDI, there are a number of core tenants. The first and most commonly stressed is obtaining the "critical view of safety" (Fig. 6.1). This concept mandates that the fundus of the gallbladder be retracted superiorly while the infundibulum is retracted laterally. This exposure generally allows the surgeon to carefully dissect out the triangle of Calot leaving only two structures connected to the lower end of the gallbladder: the cystic artery and cystic duct. The critical view of safety has also been enhanced to now describe both anterior and posterior views (Fig. 6.2). While this maneuver is the single most effective means of preventing a BDI, the reality is substantially more complex. In scenarios of a short or nonexistent cystic duct, or a small common bile duct (common in AC), these structures can be confused for each other. Furthermore, inappropriate or overzealous traction then makes these associations even more challenging. Similarly, inflammation closes the space between the gallbladder and the bile duct. In extreme cases, they may even be fused and move as a single unit (Mirizzi type A). This not uncommon reality makes identification of associated regional anatomy even more important for the surgeon in an attempt to orient the critical structures of interest and proceed with a safe procedure. These spatial-regional issues can be further challenged by a loss of perspective given the tendency of many camera operators to move ever closer to the operative dissection itself.

In all laparoscopic cholecystectomies for AC, the surgeon should perform a "bile duct time-out" to evaluate their understanding of targeted anatomy based on regional structures (Table 6.2). After a wide laparoscopic view of the subhepatic

space is obtained, the surgeon must lift the liver off the porta hepatis and identify a checklist of landmarks around the gallbladder, including duodenum, sulcus of Rouviere, umbilical fissure, pulsations of the common hepatic artery, and the bile duct itself. Once these landmarks are identified, a careful dissection of the triangle of Calot can be accomplished with minimal cautery. A specific search for a sectoral duct should also be completed. Then with a cleared triangle and the true gallbladder cystic duct angle identified, the correct "cognitive map" of the biliary tree can be superimposed on the patient's specific anatomy in the correct location. In cases of severe AC, it may be unclear if the operator can safely even obtain this anatomical viewpoint (and therefore the ability to safely proceed with a laparoscopic technique). In most scenarios, however, if the surgeon can still obtain a clear dissection of the junction between the cystic duct and the gallbladder on the lateral edge, then it is safe to continue. Initial dissection in the lateral tissues for cases of a severely inflamed field is also safest from a BDI point of view. If it is unsafe to proceed with further dissection medial to the gallbladder, however, a subtotal cholecystectomy may represent the best option. The gallbladder should be opened, all stones and debris extracted, and then closed using the surgeon's preferred minimally invasive modality (endoloops, suturing, thick stapler) as long as it is safe given the regional inflammation.

During the entire operation, a surgeon must maintain a vigilant attitude and when ambiguity arises must slow down and back out the camera to widen the view of all landmarks (complete another "bile duct time-out"). The surgeon must avoid both physical and mental "tunnel visions." Inability to accurately place the cognitive map is a stop signal. If this cannot be resolved, conversion to open surgery with top-down dissection will improve safety. For patients with inflammatory obliteration of the triangle of Calot, near-total cholecystectomy or cholecystostomy can prevent injury. Furthermore, any dissection on the left side of the bile duct should be considered a "near miss." Surgeons must also have several "cognitive maps" in their minds – normal, caudal sectoral duct, and short cystic duct. The maps must be somewhat "plastic" as size, and distances vary with each patient. There may also be circumstances where no preexisting map exists (left-sided gallbladder).

The concept of performing an operative cholangiogram to demonstrate the patient's biliary anatomy and visually confirm the correct operator's map on the overlying tissue is compelling. Unfortunately this has not proven to be true in clinical practice. More specifically, the role of *routine* intraoperative cholangiography has been evaluated in patients undergoing elective cholecystectomy. Eight randomized trials (1715 patients) were analyzed in a recent systematic review without showing any clear evidence to support its routine use. An even more recent Medicare-based study

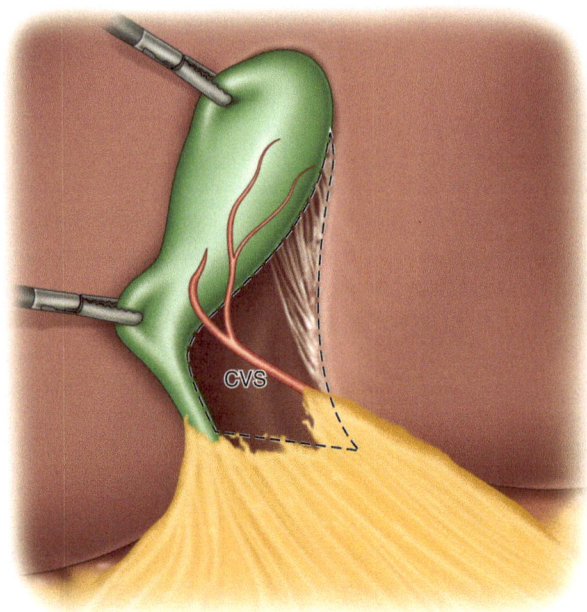

Fig. 6.1 Critical view of safety

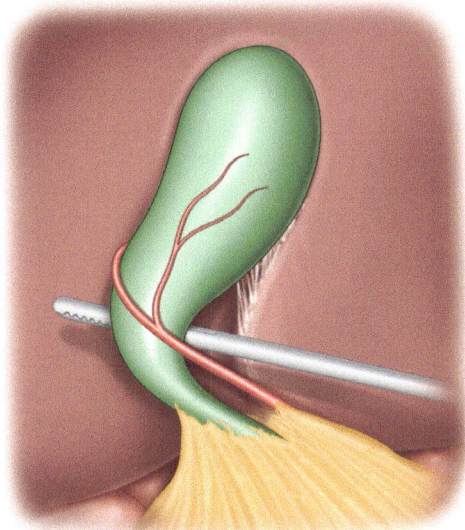
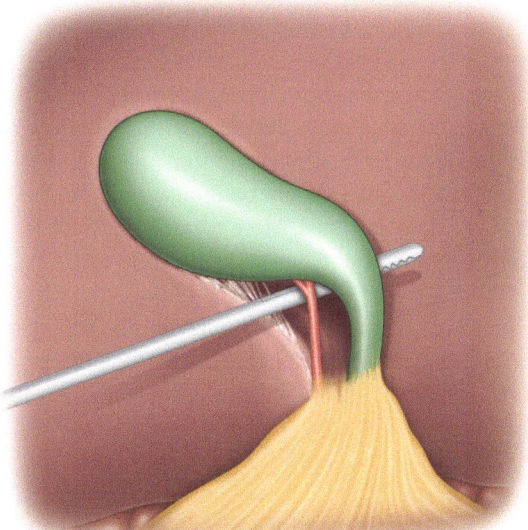

Anterior view   **Posterior view**

Fig. 6.2 Enhanced critical view of safety

Table 6.2 Bile duct "time-out" (B.E. S.A.F.E.)

B – bile duct
E – enteric (duodenum) position
S – sulcus of Rouviere
A – artery (hepatic artery)
F – fissure (umbilical fissure)
E – environment (back the camera out for improved perspective)

analyzing over 92000 patients undergoing cholecystectomy identified no statistically significant association between intraoperative cholangiography and BDI. The authors therefore concluded that intraoperative cholangiography is not effective as a preventive strategy against BDI during cholecystectomy. When this is combined with the fact that there are no randomized studies in patients undergoing cholecystectomy for AC, intraoperative cholangiography should be performed selectively in the setting of concerning pre- and/or intraoperative findings.

Postoperative Concerns

The dominant concern in the postoperative period remains a BDI. These can lead to either postoperative biliary leaks/bilomas or strictures. Although a detailed description of BDI and their reconstructions is beyond the scope of this review, it is important to consider this diagnosis, as the ACS surgeon is often called as the initial consultant by a surgeon in need. Based on large population studies, the rate of BDI approaches 0.4% using laparoscopic techniques and 0.1% with open approaches. Most BDIs are not recognized intra-

operatively, and instead patients return to the hospital with complaints of nausea, vomiting, abdominal discomfort, and potentially obstructive biliary symptoms. The ACS surgeon must hold diagnoses of a BDI and/or biloma high in their differential diagnosis when assessing these postoperative patients. Liver function tests may be abnormally elevated not only due to obstruction but also because of a biloma. These patients should be studied immediately with an abdominal US and/or CT to define the presence of collections or abnormal free fluid. It is important to note that the absence of fluid does not exclude the occurrence of a BDI. Any fluid collection should be drained with a percutaneous approach. The biliary tree, and specifically the level of injury, may then be defined with an MRC and/or ERCP. In scenarios where the posterior sector has been isolated or there has been a complete common ductal transection, retrograde drain cholangiograms and/or percutaneous transhepatic cholangiograms (and catheters) are required, respectively. It should be noted that in all BDI patients, causes of acute sepsis may be multifold: (1) intra-abdominal collections/biloma (usually related to the gallbladder bed), (2) biliperitoneum, (3) cholangitis (when the bile duct has been completely transected and clipped), and (4) liver necrosis/failure when the BDI is associated with a vascular injury. Since the specific cause of sepsis is usually unknown at the time of presentation, all critically ill patients should receive immediate fluid resuscitation and antibiotics. Blood and intra-abdominal cultures are mandatory to guide the therapy.

It should also be noted that if a BDI is suspected (extensive inflammation, severely contracted gallbladders, unexpected bleeding that requires multiple clips for control, abnormal anatomy, bile within the operative field, or difficulty in defining the triangle of Calot, sulcus of Rouviere, and critical view of safety) and/or identified within the intraoperative setting, the surgeon should consider *not* repairing the injury and risk further complicating the situation. The biliary tree/subhepatic space should be drained widely, but the bile duct should not be ligated. More specifically, ligation of the proximal bile duct stump most often leads to necrosis, subsequent bile leakage, and a more challenging reconstruction due to proximal migration of the injury itself. Prompt transfer to a tertiary hepatobiliary center should then be pursued. There is overwhelming evidence that patients display superior outcomes and long-term quality of life scores when BDIs are reconstructed by high-volume hepatobiliary surgeons. Considerations such as concurrent vasculobiliary trauma, integrity of the hilar arterial plexus, and posterior sectoral bile duct injuries are generally best appreciated in experienced centers (Table 6.2).

Additional Technical Tips for the Management of the Difficult Gallbladder

Despite all of the preceding advice and experience, there are gallbladders we each encounter that remain extremely challenging and potentially dangerous because of incredibly dense inflammation within the porta hepatis. If the operator cannot define the lateral junction between the cystic duct and the gallbladder pouch as one of their earliest maneuvers, it is generally considered unsafe to proceed with medial dissection of the triangle of Calot because the critical view is rarely attainable. This scenario should mandate one of two responses: (1) conversion to an open procedure *if* the operator has sufficient experience and training in performing the open technique or (2) placement of soft rubber tube within the inflamed gallbladder fundus to achieve decompression and therefore temporize the acute situation. This second maneuver allows the surgeon to consult and/or transfer the patient to a more experienced biliary surgeon at his/her discretion. The only other safe solution remains immediate removal of the laparoscope without any additional intervention. This mandates *immediate* transfer of the patient to a more experienced colleague and remains a reasonable response. It is clearly preferable to wander into the triangle/ porta and create a bile duct injury and/or significant hemorrhage.

Additional technical tips include draining the gallbladder early when presented with a tense and/or thickened/inflamed gallbladder wall prior to attempts at traction and dissection. In the setting of a severely thickened gallbladder wall, the operator can grasp the outside wall with one side of the grasper and the inside wall with the other (i.e., through the actual decompression hole). The authors have yet to experience a scenario outside of gallbladder cancer where this technique is not helpful. If the operator identifies a severely inflamed gallbladder that is absolutely adherent and not easily separated from either the colon or duodenum, then it should elicit a response similar to the inflamed porta hepatis as described above. More specifically, it is better to decompress the gallbladder with a tube cholecystostomy than proceed with creating an unplanned hole in the colon or duodenum. If a cholecystoduodenal fistula is suspected, however, the surgeon is advised to open the gallbladder fundus, remove all stones, and ideally perform a subtotal cholecystectomy. This can be achieved using either an open or laparoscopic technique depending on operator experience and comfort. It also removes the direct pressure caused by the impacted stone(s) and almost always allows spontaneous closure of the fistula over time. In the unusual scenario of a patient having subsequent and/or persistent issues with the remnant gallbladder, an elective completion cholecystectomy can be performed in a much more controlled and safe manner at a later date. It should also be noted that subtotal or partial cholecystectomies can be employed for a number of indications that surround two core principles. The first is a lack of surgeon comfort/experience with proceeding toward a severely inflamed porta hepatis in general. The second is a bailout maneuver in the context of a Mirizzi's syndrome. More specifically, few acute care surgeons will be comfortable in separating a contracted gallbladder from an adherent bile duct (Mirizzi type A). This is even more important when a true fistula (as opposed to simple adherence) is present between the gallbladder and the common bile duct (Mirizzi type B). In any surgical exploration of a suspected Mirizzi type B, the surgeon should be prepared to divide the common bile duct and perform a Roux-en-Y hepaticojejunostomy if required. As a result, the surprise encounter of Mirizzi anatomy during a cholecystectomy should initiate opening the gallbladder fundus, removing all stones, and proceeding with a subtotal cholecystectomy. (Fig. 6.3) Closure of the gallbladder itself can be achieved via sutures and occasionally endoscopic staplers or suture loops depending on the thickness of the gallbladder wall and staple options.

Hydrodissection utilizing a suction/irrigation catheter can be extremely helpful in the dissection of the inflamed gallbladder, triangle of Calot, and/or porta hepatis. This technique demands a steady hand and short intentional repetitive movements. While other surgeons more commonly utilize sharp Metzenbaum dissection (vs. cautery), each technique can be both safe and unsafe in the right or wrong surgical hands, respectively. Clearly one advantage of both the suction and sharp dissection, however, is the lack of concern regarding electrocautery injuries/jumping to the common bile duct.

Fig. 6.3 Mirizzi syndrome and cholecystobiliary fistula (Adapted from A. Csendes, et al.)

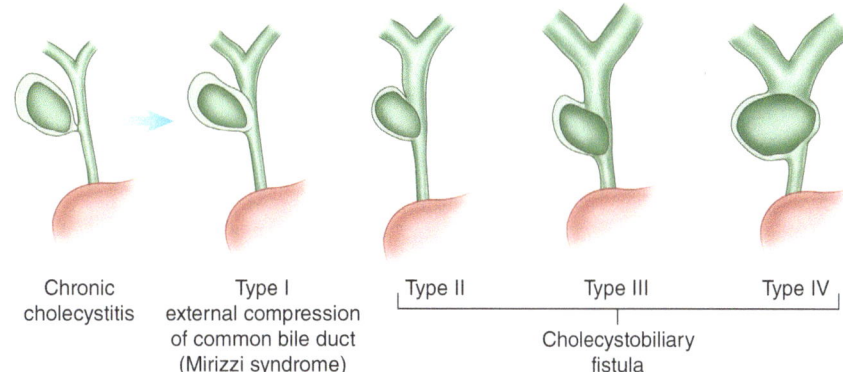

Chronic cholecystitis | Type I external compression of common bile duct (Mirizzi syndrome) | Type II   Type III   Type IV Cholecystobiliary fistula

When the surgeon identifies bile-stained tissues during their dissection in the context of a non-perforated gallbladder, concern for an unrecognized bile duct injury must be at the top of the differential diagnosis. Given the lack of current comfort in performing open explorations, most advanced biliary surgeons would recommend simple closed suction drainage of the area and prompt referral. Subsequent diagnostic evaluations may include MRCP, HIDA, ERCP, and/or tube cholangiograms. The guiding principle is to elicit no additional harm, control the bile leak, prevent sepsis, and refer the patient to a biliary expert. The role of intraoperative cholangiograms (IOC) also remains very controversial. While any potential benefit of *routine* IOC in preventing bile duct injuries has been debunked, the role of *on-demand* IOCs when the surgeon has an anatomical concern is less clear. More specifically, over 50% of IOCs are misinterpreted by the operating surgeon. As a result, the very utility of IOCs, even in times of intraoperative confusion, is unclear. If the surgeon performs an IOC, however, complete filling of all three sectors of the liver is essential to rule out segmental or sectoral bile duct injuries (e.g., transection and subsequent disconnection of low-inserting posterior sectoral ducts).

Significant hemorrhage from the gallbladder fossa/liver bed is typically a direct result of injuring the superficial branch of the middle hepatic vein. This high-flow branch is found directly adherent and/or within 1 mm of the deep gallbladder wall in 20% of all patients. When this hemorrhage occurs, the surgeon must have a defined algorithm of technical maneuvers ready to apply. Assuming this bleeding is truly from the gallbladder fossa (i.e., away from the porta hepatis), our authors typically apply precision hook electrocautery at a high setting (100 spray coagulation) directly to the site of bleeding. Persistent attempts at applying low-voltage cautery often leads to flailing and deeper dissection of the venous branch with an *increase* in the rate of bleeding. If this technique fails, place a large clip directly into the liver parenchyma at a perpendicular angle to the site of bleeding. Proceed to ignite the clip with electrocautery. This technique is used in open hepatic surgery and allows a deeper burn

along the bleeding vein. If these two techniques are insufficient (extremely rare), sponges should be packed into the adjacent space, and rapid conversion to an open procedure must be achieved. Similar to elective resections for cirrhotic patients, it is also helpful to dramatically increase the insufflation pressure within the peritoneal cavity to assist in the tamponade of low-pressure venous bleeding.

The acute care surgeon should be liberal in their use of the local/regional hepatobiliary referral service. All areas in North America now have access to high-volume HPB referral centers with subspecialty surgeons experienced in advanced hepatobiliary surgery and complication management. In most cities this service is on call at all times and may in fact travel to the referring center to assist in repairing/reconstructing biliary injuries in particular. Similar to a modern trauma service/system, HPB services should be accessible and helpful in times of need.

Take-Home Messages

1. The standard of care for acute cholecystitis remains early laparoscopic cholecystectomy.
2. The operator must identify the critical view of safety prior to ligating any structures during a laparoscopic cholecystectomy.
3. The operator should perform a bile duct time-out using the B.E. S.A.F.E. methodology prior to ligating any structures during a laparoscopic cholecystectomy.
4. Intraoperative bile duct injuries mandate experienced assistance for reconstruction. Drainage, closure and transfer to a high volume hepatobiliary service is then mandatory.
5. Patients who return with symptoms not consistent with the normal evolution of post-laparoscopic cholecystectomy should undergo immediate ultrasound or CT imaging and drainage of any fluid collection(s).

Key References

1. Yokoe M, Takada T, Strasberg SM, Solomkin JS, Mayumi T, Gomi H, et al. New diagnostic criteria and severity assessment of acute cholecystitis in revised Tokyo guidelines. J Hepatobiliary Pancreat Sci. 2012;19(5):578–85.
2. Yamashita Y, Takada T, Kawarada Y, Nimura Y, Hirota M, Miura F, et al. Surgical treatment of patients with acute cholecystitis: Tokyo guidelines. J Hepato-Biliary-Pancreat Surg. 2007;14(1):91–7.
3. Gutt CN, Encke J, Koninger J, Harnoss JC, Weigand K, Kipfmuller K, et al. Acute cholecystitis: early versus delayed cholecystectomy, a multicenter randomized trial (ACDC study, NCT00447304). Ann Surg. 2013;258(3):385–93.
4. Way LW, Stewart L, Gantert W, et al. Causes and prevention of laparoscopic bile duct injuries: analysis of 252 cases from a human factors and cognitive psychology perspective. Ann Surg. 2003;273:460.
5. Sheffield KM, Riall TS, Kuo YF, et al. Association between cholecystectomy with vs. without intraoperative cholangiography and risk of common duct injury. JAMA. 2013;310:812.

Minimally Invasive Approach to Choledocholithiasis

Caolan Walsh, Amy Neville, Diederick Jalink, and Fady K. Balaa

Introduction

The prevalence of gallstones in the United States is estimated to be 7–10%; however only a minority of patients with asymptomatic gallstones will ever become symptomatic [1]. The prevalence of common bile duct stones, also referred to as choledocholithiaisis, may be seen in 10–15% of patients with gallstones [2]. Evaluating and treating calculous disease of the bile duct have been well described [3]. Biliary tract disease is significantly more prevalent in the morbidly obese patient and has been reported as high as 45% [4]. Patients undergoing weight loss surgery are at increased risk of developing gallstones or sludge. Serial postoperative ultrasounds have demonstrated 30–36% of patients, who were previously stone-free, will develop cholelithiasis within the first year after surgery [5]. The incidence of bariatric surgery continues to rise, and according to the most recent estimates by the American Society for Metabolic and Bariatric Surgery, more than 200,000 bariatric procedures are being performed annually in the United States. Approximately one quarter of these procedures are Roux-en-Y gastric bypass; therefore at the current volumes, as many as five hundred thousand individuals per decade will have bypass anatomy. Although the true incidence of symptomatic choledocholithiasis in patients following gastric bypass is not known, some series have reported a very low incidence (0.4%) over 6 years [6]. Managing common bile duct stones in patients post gastric bypass poses particular anatomical barriers and challenges. Despite these challenges, the vast majority of patients with bypass anatomy are managed with a minimally invasive approach. This chapter will discuss the pathophysiology, prevention, clinical manifestation, diagnosis, and surgical treatment of choledocholithiasis with a focus on patients with gastric bypass anatomy.

Pathophysiology

The liver produces approximately 500–1000 mL of bile per day. The gallbladder will typically contain 50–100 mL of concentrated bile at any given time. Water excluded, bile is composed of bile salts, fatty acids, cholesterol, protein, bilirubin, phospholipids, and other trace elements. Cholesterol stones are composed of crystalline cholesterol monohydrate, are formed within gallbladder, and are generally soft. Bilirubin stones, also known as pigment stones, are formed by bilirubin calcium salts and typically materialize in the common bile duct. In North America, common bile duct stones are predominantly cholesterol stones that have migrated from the gallbladder. In Asia, pigmented stones make up the majority of common bile duct stones. Cholesterol is rendered soluble in bile by the effects of hydrophilic bile salts and lipophilic lecithins. When the solubilizing capacity of bile is overwhelmed by cholesterol, the excess will aggregate into crystals. Obesity will cause an increased hepatic cholesterol secretion; however bile salt secretions remain largely unchanged. The amount of cholesterol secreted into bile has a linear relationship with total body weight [7]. Weight loss is associated with a reduction of bile salt pool and increases mobilization of adipose tissue and cholesterol therefore increasing the rates of gallstones.

C. Walsh (✉)
The Ottawa Hospital, Department of General Surgery, Ottawa, ON, Canada
e-mail: caowalsh@toh.ca

A. Neville
The Ottawa Hospital, University of Ottawa, Department of Surgery, Ottawa, ON, Canada

D. Jalink
Kingston Health Sciences Centre, Department of General Surgery, Kingston, ON, Canada

F.K. Balaa
The Ottawa Hospital, The Ottawa Hospital, General Campus, Ottawa, ON, Canada

© Springer International Publishing AG 2018
K.A. Khwaja, J.J. Diaz (eds.), *Minimally Invasive Acute Care Surgery*, https://doi.org/10.1007/978-3-319-64723-4_7

Prevention

There are two strategies for gallstone prevention after a bypass operation: prophylactic cholecystectomy and pharmacotherapy. Concomitant cholecystectomy was a common practice in the era of open Roux-en-Y gastric bypass [8]. Even without evidence of preoperative cholelithiasis, the high incidence of postoperative gallstone or sludge formation was reason enough for most surgeons to perform a concomitant cholecystectomy given the difficulty of reoperation in this patient population. Today, over 95% of gastric bypass operations are performed laparoscopically. Performing a cholecystectomy at the same time as the gastric bypass has been shown to significantly increase operative time and double the hospital stay [9]. Although some series show a high incidence symptomatic cholelithiasis of 15.6% after gastric bypass, most series confirm only the minority of patients will ever develop symptoms (1.4–5.4%) [10, 11]. Therefore, a more common practice is the removal of the gallbladder only in symptomatic patients with evidence of cholelithiasis.

Pharmacologic prophylaxis has also been proven effective. A 6-month course of ursodiol 600 mg daily following surgery has been shown to significantly reduce the incidence of gallstone formation from 32 to 2% [12]. Unfortunately, the high cost and side effects of this drug have generally resulted in low compliance [12, 13].

Clinical Manifestation

Acute obstruction of the bile duct by a stone causes a rapid distension of the biliary tree and activation of local pain fibers. Pain is the most common presenting symptom for choledocholithiasis and is localized to either the right upper quadrant or to the epigastrium. The obstruction will also cause bile stasis which is a risk factor for bacterial overgrowth. The bacteria may originate from the duodenum or the stone itself. The combination of biliary obstruction and colonization of the biliary tree will lead to the development of fevers, the second most common presenting symptom of choledocholithiasis. Biliary obstruction, if unrelieved, will lead to jaundice. When these three symptoms (pain, fever, and jaundice) are found simultaneously, it is known as Charcot's triad. This triad suggests the diagnosis of acute ascending cholangitis, a potentially life-threatening condition. If not treated promptly, this can lead to hypotension and decreased metal status, both signs of severe sepsis. When combined with Charcot's triad, this constellation of symptoms is commonly referred to as Reynolds pentad.

Diagnosis

The diagnosis of choledocholithiasis should be made with the combined information found with clinical findings, laboratory results, and radiology. Fever, nausea, and right upper quadrant pain may all be present in similar frequencies in gallstones and common duct stones. Jaundice, pruritus, and dark urine are much more frequent in common duct stones compared to gallstones [14].

Ultrasound is a fast, noninvasive, and relatively inexpensive modality for assessing biliary anatomy; however it may not always be able to identify small or distal common bile duct stones (Fig. 7.1). Magnetic retrograde cholangiopancreatography (MRCP) is highly sensitive (90–100%) and highly specific (88–96%) for the diagnosis of choledocholithiasis. In one study, sensitivity and specificity were 100% and 99%, respectively, for stones ≥7 mm [15, 16]. In an asymptomatic or stable patient, MRCP should be used to confirm the presence of a common bile duct stone. Potential drawbacks of MRCP include cost and availability. Furthermore, this investigation is purely diagnostic and cannot deliver therapy. Endoscopic retrograde cholangiopancreatography (ERCP) is a highly sensitive and specific diagnostic modality for common duct stones and can also be therapeutic. In a gastric bypass patient, ERCP can be technically complex. The ampulla can be reached in two ways: with the peroral technique by navigating the scope through the alimentary and biliary limbs of small bowel or through an operative, transgastric approach. Some institutions have reported success rates as high as 90% in reaching the ampulla and 80% successful in delivering therapy to the common bile duct in gastric bypass patients using peroral ERCP [17].

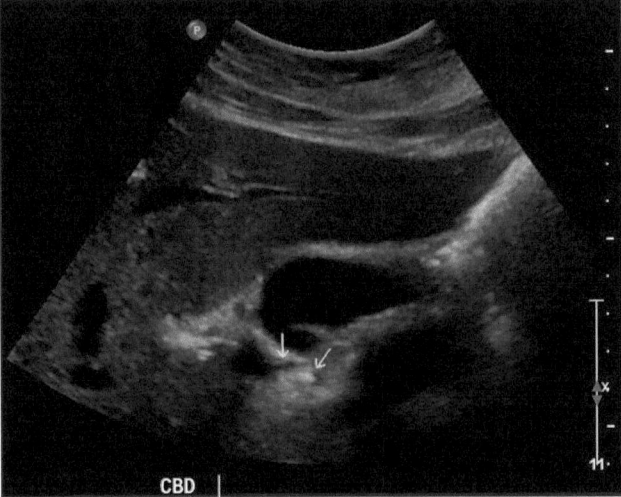

Fig. 7.1 Ultrasound identification of common bile duct stones

These numbers, although impressive, do not likely represent the success rates of the majority of centers. Given the invasiveness of ERCP in a gastric bypass patient, ERCP should be reserved for therapeutic purposes only and is not an appropriate diagnostic test in the majority of cases.

Management

The management of choledocholithiasis in a patient with previous gastric bypass must include a multidisciplinary team approach and must take into consideration local expertise and availability of resources. Factors to consider in designing a treatment plan include the clinical stability of the patient, the alimentary and biliary limb length if the operative report is available, the size of the common duct, and the size and location of the stone. If present, how to manage the gallbladder itself must also factor into the decision. Once the diagnosis is confirmed, potential management options include endoscopic and/or operative therapy.

Asymptomatic or minimally symptomatic patients with common duct stones and concomitant in situ gallbladder can be managed with simultaneous laparoscopic cholecystectomy and either transgastric ERCP or bile duct exploration. In centers with adequate experience and training in advanced endoscopy, peroral ERCP may be considered initially, followed by laparoscopic cholecystectomy. In individuals with biliary pancreatitis, a cholangiogram should be performed at the same time as the laparoscopic cholecystectomy. If positive, an intraoperative transgastric ERCP or laparoscopic common bile duct exploration should be performed. In patients with signs of acute ascending cholangitis, administration of intravenous

fluids and antibiotics is crucial. In the rare event the sepsis cannot be controlled with the appropriate antibiotics, a radiologically placed biliary decompression drain should be strongly considered until definitive therapy can be arranged. If radiology is unsuccessful, surgical drainage of the common bile duct with a T-tube is performed, and definitive stone management is deferred. Retained stones with previous common bile duct exploration may be managed by interventional radiology if a T-tube is present. Referral to hepatobiliary surgery should be considered in the event of impacted stone at the ampulla or multiple intrahepatic stones. In these scenarios, therapy will likely require more complex biliary manipulation, reconstruction, or hepatic resection (Table 7.1).

Endoscopic Therapy

Endoscopic retrograde cholangiopancreatography (ERCP) may be considered depending on the availability and experience of an advanced endoscopist. To successfully complete an ERCP in a gastric bypass patient, a long enteroscope must successfully travel down the Roux limb, navigate the jejunojejunostomy, and travel back up the biliary limb to the second stage of the duodenum. Many different types of scopes can be utilized with a wide range of scope lengths, thicknesses, balloons, and viewing angles; the specific technical description is beyond the scope of this chapter. Predictors of endoscopic success include the patients who have a short biliopancreatic limb ($\leq$50 cm) and short alimentary limb ($\leq$100 cm). Potential complications of the ERCP in this specific clinical circumstance include failed intervention, perforation, bleeding, and pancreatitis.

Table 7.1 Procedural intervention options in different clinical scenarios

Clinical scenario	Therapeutic options
Incidental choledocholithiasis or obstructive jaundice (gallbladder present)	Laparoscopic cholecystectomy + LCBDE/OCBDE Laparoscopic cholecystectomy + IO ERCPPeroral ERCP followed by laparoscopic cholecystectomy
Incidental choledocholithiasis or obstructive jaundice (gallbladder absent)	Peroral ERCPIO ERCP LCBDE/OCBDE
Biliary pancreatitis	Laparoscopic cholecystectomy with IOC *If IOC positive* IO ERCP or LCBDE/OCBDE
Ascending cholangitis (despite IV fluids and IV antibiotics)	Percutaneous transhepatic drainageLaparoscopic or open placement of T-tube
Retained stone after duct exploration	If T-tube in place: IR If no T-tube: IO ERCP

Impacted stone in the ampulla
Multiple intrahepatic stones
	Referral to hepatobiliary surgery*Dilated duct*
	  Choledochoduodenostomy Hepaticojejunostomy*Non-dilated duct*
	  Transduodenal sphincteroplasty

ERCP endoscopic retrograde cholangiopancreatography, *LCBDE* laparoscopic common bile duct exploration, *OCBDE* open common bile duct exploration, *IO* intraoperative, *IOC* intraoperative cholangiogram, *IR* interventional radiology

Operative Therapy

When planning a surgical intervention, it is essential to know the size and location of the stone(s), the size of the common bile duct, and whether the gallbladder is present. Surgical options for addressing choledocholithiasis following gastric bypass include laparoscopic-assisted transgastric ERCP, laparoscopic common bile duct exploration, and open common bile duct exploration.

Laparoscopic Common Bile Duct Exploration

Laparoscopic Intraoperative Cholangiogram

The patient, surgeon, assistant, and equipment position can be seen in Fig. 7.2. The port placement can be seen in Fig. 7.3. The gallbladder and structures of the hepatocystic triangle should be dissected free as with performing a standard laparoscopic cholecystectomy. Once the critical view of safety

Fig. 7.2 Operative room setup

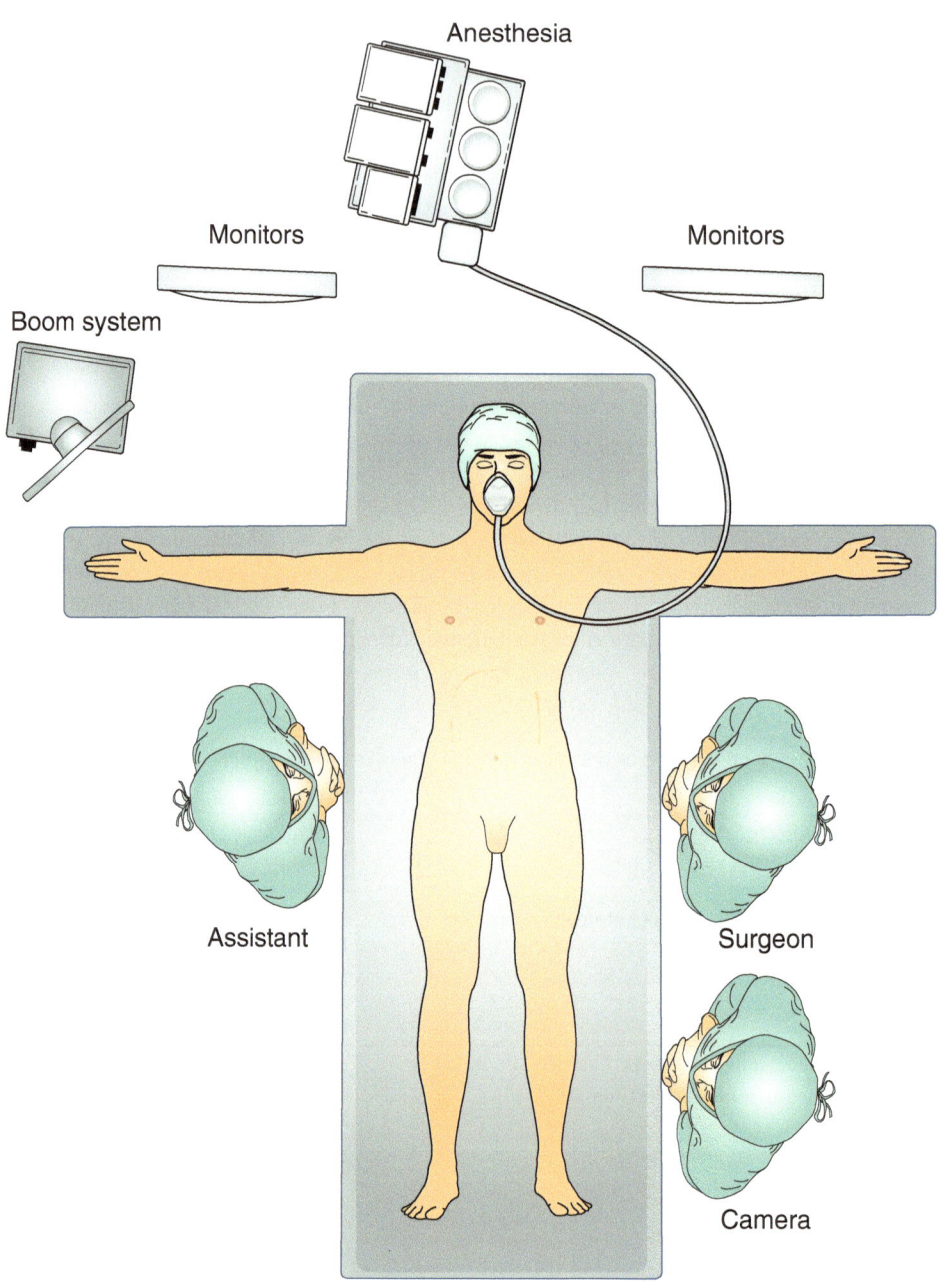

Fig. 7.3 Trocar placement

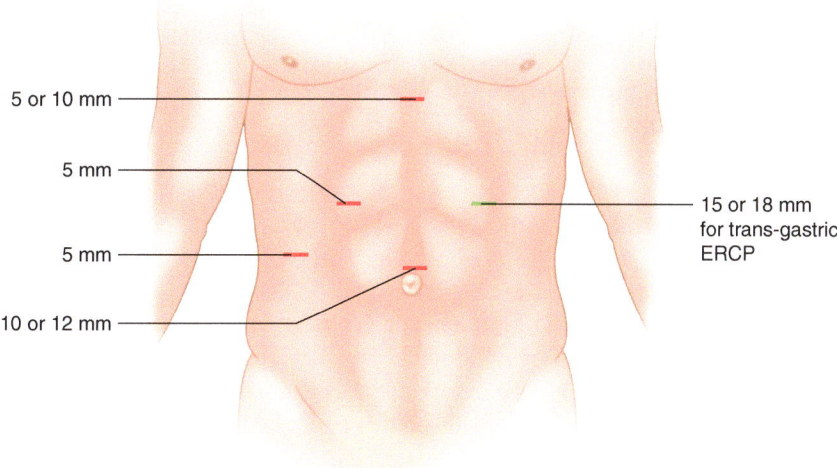

5 or 10 mm

5 mm

5 mm

10 or 12 mm

15 or 18 mm
for trans-gastric
ERCP

is obtained, a single clip is placed close to the gallbladder, and the cystic duct is sharply cut with Metzenbaum scissors, no more than half its circumference. A cholangiogram catheter is passed into the abdomen through one of the right subcostal ports with the Olsen-Reddick cholangiogram clamp or through a separate incision with an introducer sheath. The catheter should be positioned in line with the cystic duct to allow easier entry. The tip of the catheter is guided into the cystic duct and secured in place with a clamp or a metal clip. If the cystic duct is not easily identifiable, a small incision in the infundibulum of the gallbladder may be performed and insertion of the cholangiogram catheter via the gallbladder (transcholecystic). This technique is more difficult and can lead to spilling of large quantities of bile or stones. In this circumstance, the use of an EndoLoop™ around the gallbladder may assist in getting an adequate seal around the catheter and prevent leaking of contrast. Prior to performing the cholangiogram, it is imperative to ensure the system is free of all air bubble. Numerous contrast agents are available; the contrast used at our institution is Isovue-300™ (Iopamidol Injection 61%, NDC 0270–1315) full strength or mixed 50:50 with saline. The patient is placed in the Trendelenberg position, and the first injection is performed. A satisfactory cholangiogram must visualize the left and right anterior and posterior hepatic ducts as well as show contrast entering the duodenum. Changes in patient positioning, including placing the patient in reverse Trendelenberg position to visualize the duodenum, may be necessary. Small stones (≤4 mm) may be flushed through the ampulla with administration of glucagon 1 g IV and flushing the common

bile duct with saline. If this is successful, a final cholangiogram should be performed to confirm the absence of any residual stones or debris.

Laparoscopic Common Bile Duct Exploration

This procedure can further be divided into two subcategories: transcystic/transcholecystic and choledochotomy. The transcystic and transcholecystic approach are appropriate for stones ≤10 mm in size and located distal to the cystic duct takeoff. A choledochotomy is typically reserved for patients with a common bile duct ≥10 mm and will allow retrieval of stones ≥10 mm in size or stones proximal to the cystic duct takeoff.

Laparoscopic Common Bile Duct Exploration: Transcystic/Transcholecystic

Once the cholangiogram is complete, a guide wire is fed into the CBD. The cystic duct is dilated with a balloon catheter up to the size of the largest known stone. Typically, the cystic duct is not dilated more than the size of the CBD or to a maximum of 10 mm. Removal of the stone can be performed in a retrograde fashion with a basket or in an antegrade fashion with a balloon. If the retrograde technique is used, a choledochoscope can be used to visualize, grasp, and retrieve the stone. For the antegrade technique, the ampulla is dilated with a balloon, and the stones are pushed into the duodenum. This technique can be complicated by bleeding and pancreatitis.

Once completed, a final cholangiogram should be performed to confirm the absence of residual stones or ductal leak. The cystic duct is ligated with clips or an EndoLoop™.

Laparoscopic Common Bile Duct Exploration: Choledochotomy

This technique may be required in the patient with a previous cholecystectomy, failed or difficult transcystic approach, or retrieving stones proximal to the cystic duct takeoff. The porta is carefully dissected until the identification of the anterior surface of the CBD. Confirmation can be achieved by fine needle aspiration or ultrasound. Two lateral stay sutures are placed on the distal common bile duct to aid with retraction. A longitudinal choledochotomy is performed on the anterior wall of the CBD with Metzenbaum scissors. Lateral deviation or a transverse incision may compromise the blood supply of the CBD and should be avoided. The length of the incision should be no longer than the size of the largest known stone. Similar to the transcystic approach, a catheter is placed through one of the laparoscopic ports or through a separate skin incision. The epigastric port is often used since its position allows for easier placement of the catheter into the CBD. Glucagon IV is administered and the catheter is now flushed with saline. This first step may be all that is required to clear the duct of small stones. If the stone remains, exploration is similar to the transcystic approach mentioned above. A final cholangiogram should always be performed before terminating the procedure. The common duct can be closed primarily with 5–0 PDS. Closure over a T-tube should be considered in the presence of residual stones, a concern of stricture, or the required access to the biliary system postoperatively.

Laparoscopic Gastrotomy and Intraoperative ERCP

In patients with a small common bile duct (≤10 mm) and small stones (≤10 mm), a laparoscopic-assisted ERCP may also be considered. The ports, assistant, and surgeons' position should be unchanged from a non-bypass patient. The standard ports at our institution are a 10 mm supraumbilical port, a 5 or 10 mm subxiphoid port, and two 5 mm right subcostal ports. After the cholecystectomy is performed, an additional 15 mm or 18 mm port is placed in the left upper quadrant (LUQ). Lysis of adhesions might be required to better visualize the remnant stomach. A purse-string suture with an absorbable suture (e.g., #1 Vicryl) is placed in the body of the gastric remnant. A gastrostomy is performed with L-hook electrosurgery device, and the tip of the LUQ port is guided into the stomach. The purse-string suture is

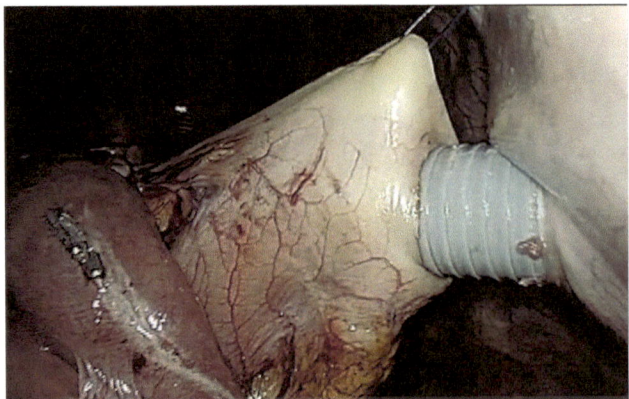

Fig. 7.4 Placement of a 15 mm trocar into the remnant stomach

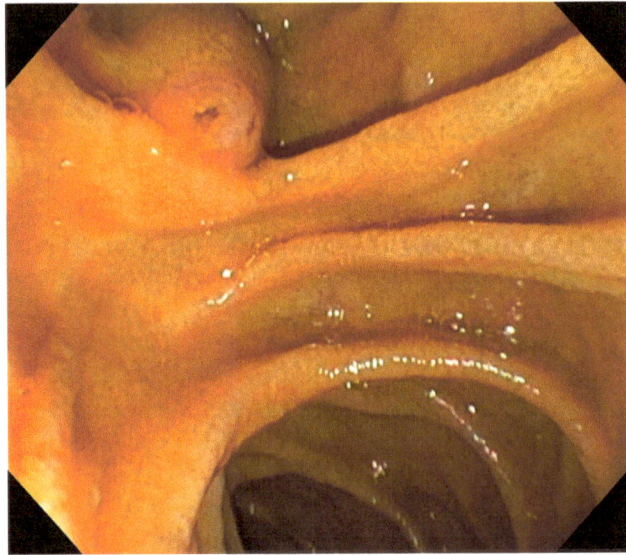

Fig. 7.5 Endoscopic visualization of the ampulla

tightened slightly to avoid leaking. Alternatively, the stomach may be elevated to the abdominal wall with a suture, and the port can be inserted through a small gastrotomy (Fig. 7.4). The side viewing duodenal scope can now be introduced through the port and into the gastric remnant. The surgeon should stabilize the scope at the level of the port while the endoscopist performs the ERCP. The identification of the ampulla is similar to a peroral ERCP (Fig. 7.5). When possible, endoscopic CO_2 should be insufflated in lieu of air. It is recommended to occlude the jejunum just distal to the ligament of Treitz with a bowel grasper to avoid gaseous distention of the small bowel and subsequent loss of laparoscopic visualization. Once successful, the scope is removed, and the gastrotomy is closed with the previously placed purse string, with separate laparoscopic sutures (Fig. 7.6) or with a laparoscopic stapler.

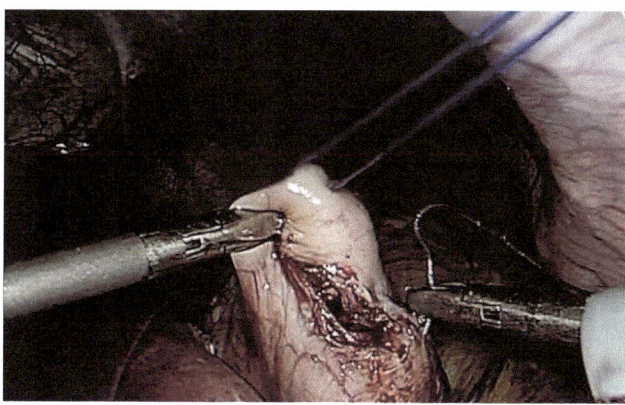

Fig. 7.6 Suture closure of the gastrotomy

Conclusions

The high incidence of gallstone disease combined with high volume of bariatric procedures currently being performed will likely lead to an increase in choledocholithiasis in gastric bypass patients. If current volumes of bariatric surgery remain constant, as many as five hundred thousand individuals in the Unites States will have Roux-en-Y gastric bypass anatomy every decade. Preventative measures by means of prophylactic cholecystectomy or pharmacology seem to have minimal role, especially since the transition from open to laparoscopic surgery. Peroral ERCP may be considered in centers with adequate expertise. Surgery remains a very valuable tool in this patient population and will likely be required in the majority of these patients.

Take-Home Messages

- As several thousand Roux-en-Y gastric bypasses are being performed annually in North America, choledocholithiasis in patients with altered gastrointestinal anatomy will be encountered by many bariatric and general surgeons.
- In the presence of Roux-en-Y gastric bypass anatomy, ERCP should not be considered a diagnostic tool. MRCP should strongly be considered in all patients with high clinical suspicion to confirm the diagnosis of choledocholithiasis.
- Surgeons, advanced endoscopists, and interventional radiologists are often required together to diagnose and treat common bile duct stones in the bypass patient.
- Although some high-volume centers may be able to treat these individuals with peroral endoscopy, the majority of cases will require a combined laparoscopic and endoscopic approach.

Key References

1. Everhart JE, Khare M, Hill M, Maurer KR. Prevalence and ethnic differences in gallbladder disease in the United States. Gastroenterology. 1999;117(3):632–9.
2. Tazuma S. Gallstone disease: epidemiology, pathogenesis, and classification of biliary stones (common bile duct and intrahepatic). Best Pract Res Clin Gastroenterol. 2006;20(6):1075–83.
3. Orenstein SB, Marks JM, Hardacre JM. Technical aspects of bile duct evaluation and exploration. Surg Clin North Am. 2014;94(2):281–96. doi:10.1016/j.suc.2013.12.002.
4. Wattchow DA, Hall JC, Whiting MJ, Bradley B, Iannos J, Watts JM. Prevalence and treatment of gall stones after gastric bypass surgery for morbid obesity. Br Med J (Clin Res Ed). 1983;286(6367):763.
5. Shiffman ML, Sugerman HJ, Kellum JM, Brewer WH, Moore EW. Gallstone formation after rapid weight loss: a prospective study in patients undergoing gastric bypass surgery for treatment of morbid obesity. Am J Gastroenterol. 1991;86(8):1000–5.
6. Tucker O, Soriano I, Szomstein S, Rosenthal R. Management of choledocholithiasis after laparoscopic Roux-en-Y gastric bypass. Surg Obes Relat Dis. 2008;4(5):674–8. doi:10.1016/j.soard.2008.01.014. Epub 2008 Jun 9.
7. Bennion LJ, Grundy SM. Effects of obesity and caloric intake on biliary lipid metabolism in man. J Clin Invest. 1975;56(4):996–1011.
8. Schmidt JH, Hocking MP, Rout WR, Woodward ER. The case for prophylactic cholecystectomy concomitant with gastric restriction for morbid obesity. Am Surg. 1988;54(5):269–72.
9. Hamad GG, Ikramuddin S, Gourash WF, Schauer PR. Elective cholecystectomy during laparoscopic Roux-en-Y gastric bypass: is it worth the wait? Obes Surg. 2003;13(1):76–81.
10. Sugerman HJ, Sugerman EL, DeMaria EJ, Kellum JM, Kennedy C, Mowery Y, Wolfe LG. Bariatric surgery for severely obese adolescents. J Gastrointest Surg. 2003;7(1):102–7. discussion 107-8.
11. Oliak D, Ballantyne GH, Davies RJ, Wasielewski A, Schmidt HJ. Short-term results of laparoscopic gastric bypass in patients with BMI > or = 60. Obes Surg. 2002;12(5):643–7.
12. Sugerman HJ, Brewer WH, Shiffman ML, Brolin RE, Fobi MA, Linner JH, MacDonald KG, MacGregor AM, Martin LF, Oram-Smith JC. A multicenter, placebo-controlled, randomized, double-blind, prospective trial of prophylactic ursodiol for the prevention of gallstone formation following gastric-bypass-induced rapid weight loss. Am J Surg. 1995;169(1):91–6. discussion 96-7.
13. Wudel LJ Jr, Wright JK, Debelak JP, Allos TM, Shyr Y, Chapman WC. Prevention of gallstone formation in morbidly obese patients undergoing rapid weight loss: results of a randomized controlled pilot study. J Surg Res. 2002;102(1):50–6.
14. Notash AY, Salimi J, Golfam F, Habibi G, Alizadeh K. Preoperative clinical and paraclinical predictors of choledocholithiasis. Hepatobiliary Pancreat Dis Int. 2008;7(3):304–7.
15. Guarise A, Baltieri S, Mainardi P, Faccioli N. Diagnostic accuracy of MRCP in choledocholithiasis. Radiol Med. 2005;109(3):239–51.
16. Kats J, Kraai M, Dijkstra AJ, Koster K, Ter Borg F, Hazenberg HJ, Eeftinck Schattenkerk M, des Plantes BG, Eddes EH. Magnetic resonance cholangiopancreaticography as a diagnostic tool for common bile duct stones: a comparison with ERCP and clinical follow-up. Dig Surg. 2003;20(1):32–7.
17. DuCoin C, Moon RC, Teixeira AF, Jawad MA. Laparoscopic choledochoduodenostomy as an alternate treatment for common bile duct stones after Roux-en-Y gastric bypass. Surg Obes Relat Dis. 2014;10(4):647–52. doi:10.1016/j.soard.2014.01.027.

Mohammed Hassan Al Mahroos and Liane S. Feldman

Introduction

Complicated peptic ulcer disease represents a serious cause of morbidity and mortality [1] Complicated peptic ulcer disease was the most common cause of death of the 11 emergency general surgical conditions included in the Global Burden of Disease Study [2]. Perforation represents a potentially lethal complication of peptic ulcer disease with a mortality rate of up to 30% and morbidity of 50% [1, 3]. It accounts for 2–20% of complicated peptic ulcer disease but 70% of ulcer related mortality [2, 4–6]. In the United States, one in every ten hospital admissions due to perforated peptic ulcer ends in death [7].

Since the introduction of proton pump inhibitors during the last quarter of the previous century, the overall incidence of peptic ulcer has dropped significantly in developed countries. Yet the epidemiological patterns of complications, including perforation, remained the same [6, 8].

Perforated peptic ulcer presents as an acute onset of progressively worsening abdominal pain, nausea, vomiting and fever. The classical finding on physical exam is generalized peritonitis. In the elderly and in immunocompromised patients, the clinical signs can be obscured which may lead to a delay in the diagnosis [3].

Although the pathophysiology of the development of peptic ulcer disease is well-understood, the reason for why some perforate while others do not is still poorly understood.

Electronic supplementary material The online version of this chapter (doi:10.1007/978-3-319-64723-4_8) contains supplementary material, which is available to authorized users.

M.H. Al Mahroos
McGill University Health Centre, Department of Surgery,
1650 Cedar Avenue, E19-125, Montreal, QC, Canada
e-mail: mohammed.almahroos@mail.mcgill.ca

L.S. Feldman (✉)
Steinberg-Bernstein Centre for Minimally Invasive Surgery and Innovation, Division of General Surgery, McGill University Health Centre, 1650 Cedar Avenue, L9-309, Montreal, QC, Canada
e-mail: liane.feldman@mcgill.ca

Risk factors predisposing to perforation include use of nonsteroidal anti-inflammatory drugs, smoking, cocaine and methamphetamines use, steroids, high-salt diet and alcohol, *Helicobacter pylori* infection and ulcer occurring in the context of the *Zollinger-Ellison* syndrome [3, 9–14].

In this chapter, we will review the diagnosis and management of perforated peptic ulcer disease with a focus on minimally invasive approach to the surgical repair.

Preoperative Diagnosis

The surgeon should have a high degree of suspicion for perforated ulcer when a patient presents with sudden onset of severe abdominal pain, nausea, vomiting, fever and peritonitis. This can rapidly progress to septic shock if the diagnosis and treatment are delayed. The differential diagnosis may include pancreatitis, ruptured abdominal aortic aneurysm and ischemic bowel, among others.

Blood Work

Blood work may show signs of infection but are not diagnostic. Complete blood count may show elevated white blood cell count, and a blood gas may reveal elevated lactate and also can assess the degree of metabolic compromise. Blood work should also help eliminate other possible diagnoses such as acute pancreatitis.

Diagnostic Imaging

Diagnostic imaging should be performed if the status of the patient allows. Unstable patients with frank peritonitis might head straight to surgery.

Chest/Abdominal X-ray Free air on an upright chest x-ray is highly suggestive of perforated viscus. The predominant causes of pneumoperitoneum on x-ray are perforated peptic ulcer and perforated diverticulitis [15]. Erect chest or abdominal x-rays are inexpensive and quick but they have a reported sensitivity of only 75% and will not help identify the source of pneumoperitoneum [3, 15, 16].

Abdominal CT Scan This is regarded as the imaging modality of choice due to high sensitivity of 98% and ability to both identify the source of pneumoperitoneum and rule out other potential diagnoses [3, 16–18]. Abdominal CT scan will reveal pneumoperitoneum or retroperitoneal air (in cases of a posterior perforation), free fluid, signs of inflammation around the perforated segment and might show leakage of contrast if given orally.

Management

In the Emergency Department

Patients with perforated peptic ulcer can quickly progress to septic shock. Early diagnosis and initiation of treatment is important in reducing the development of septic shock and mortality [3, 13]. Therefore, immediate resuscitation with intravenous fluids, intravenous proton pump inhibitor and broad-spectrum antibiotics should be started, and patients should be continually monitored. Management at this point should follow sepsis treatment guidelines. A nasogastric tube is inserted.

Surgery vs. Observation

Nonoperative Management Herman Taylor published the first case series describing nonoperative management of perforated peptic ulcer in 1946 and reported 28 cases of which 24 were discharged after successful treatment [19].

Nonoperative management of perforated peptic ulcer may be considered in selected cases where the presumption is that the perforation has sealed by itself. Nonoperative therapy should not be offered to those who present with haemodynamic instability, with generalized peritonitis or with contrast extravasation on CT scan. Patients treated with a nonoperative approach require serial abdominal examinations and vital signs monitoring to assess for any signs of progression of the disease. Proton pump inhibitors and antibiotic therapy should be initiated. In a randomized control trial published prior to the proton pump inhibitor era, over 70% of patients with a clinical diagnosis of perforated ulcer were successfully managed nonoperatively but with a high failure rate of nonoperative management in patients older than 70 years of age [20].

Operative Management Perforated peptic ulcer can be repaired using either an open or laparoscopic approach. A Cochrane review including three randomized control trials comparing laparoscopic to open repair of perforated peptic ulcer found no difference in abdominal septic complications or pulmonary complications between the two groups with one study reporting 1 day shorter hospital stay [4, 6, 21, 22]. In an analysis of the NSQIP database using case matching, the laparoscopic approach was associated with shorter hospital stay and a non-statistically significant trend towards reduced wound complications and prolonged ventilation rates [23].

The goal of laparoscopic peptic ulcer repair is no different than that of the open repair, namely, source control through sealing of the perforation and peritoneal irrigation. Laparoscopic repair is contraindicated in the following situations: simultaneous bleeding and perforation of the peptic ulcer in the unstable patient, cardiac or pulmonary contraindications to pneumoperitoneum and expected hostile or frozen abdomen [24–27].

Our approach for to laparoscopic repair of perforated peptic ulcer will be described, including instrumentation, positioning, access, repair and post-operative management.

Instruments

- Trocars:
  - 10/12 mm blunt trocar
  - 10/12 mm sharp trocar
  - 2 to 3 5 mm trocars
- 5 mm 30° laparoscope
- Liver retractor
- Laparoscopic pressurized suction irrigator
- Non-traumatic graspers
- Laparoscopic needle drivers

Positioning The patient is supine with straight split legs, as for other upper abdominal procedures. The patient is secured to the bed to enable placement in reverse Trendelenburg position. A nasogastric tube should be in place. The surgeon stands between the patient's legs and the assistant stands to the left side of the patient. The screen is positioned at the head of the table (Fig. 8.1).

Access and Exploration We use an open technique to access the peritoneal cavity at the umbilicus and insert a 10 mm blunt trocar. Carbon dioxide is used to insufflate the peritoneal cavity to a pressure of 12–15 mmHg. Two working ports are placed on either side along the mid-clavicular lines at the level of the umbilicus: a 10 mm trocar is placed along the left mid-clavicular line and 5 mm on the right side. The left 10 mm trocar is needed to introduce the sutures. Additional 5 mm trocars can be added along the right ante-

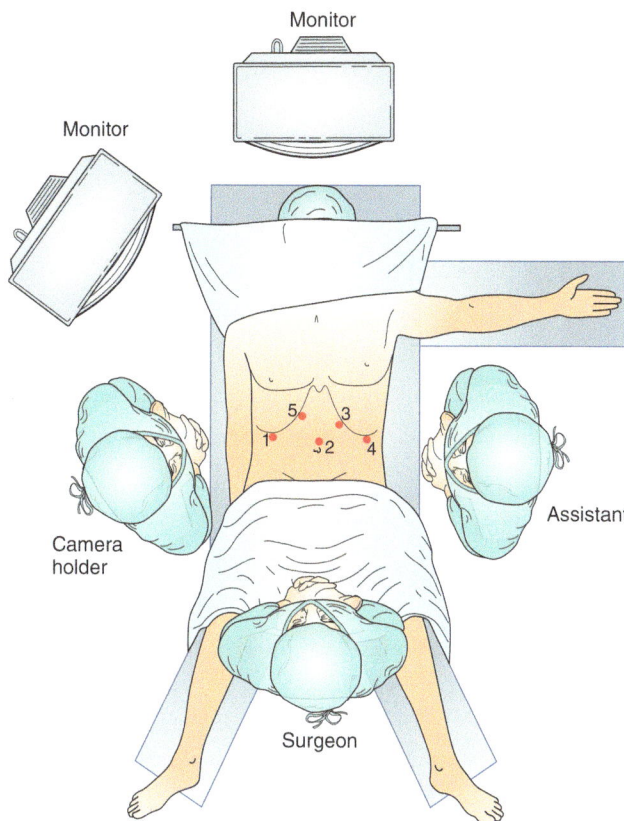

Fig. 8.1 Operating room set-up and port placement: (1) 5 mm liver retractor port, (2) 10 mm camera port, (3) 10 mm surgeon port, (4) 5 mm assistant port if needed and (5) 5 mm surgeon port [28]

rior axillary line, below the level of the liver edge, to help retract the liver. When needed, additional 5 mm trocars can be placed on the left side to be used by the assistant.

After complete examination of the peritoneal cavity, the perforation is identified after retraction of the gallbladder, which is usually adherent to the area [29].

Repair and closure The decision on the method of surgical repair of perforated peptic ulcer depends on multiple factors. While most perforations are amenable to primary closure or patch, the surgeon should consider:

- Size of the perforation: Perforations larger than 2 cm are more likely to fail primary closure or graham patch repair and might require resection [3].
- Status of the tissue: Tissues that are ischemic, necrotic or severely inflamed may preclude safe primary closure [3].
- Site of the perforation:
  - Gastric ulcers are more likely to be caused by a malignancy than duodenal ulcers. It has been reported that up to 13% of gastric perforations are due to cancer [3, 15]. Considerations for resection should be taken if the ulcer is large or the affected region has suspicious fea-

tures [3, 13, 15]. At minimum, ulcer biopsy should be performed. For ulcers in the body of the stomach, stapled resection of the ulcer can be considered. This is facilitated by placement of stay sutures in the stomach around the perforation [30].
  - Duodenal perforations can be repaired by primary closure or graham patch repair without need for biopsy.

Identification of the perforation

- As most perforations are around the pyloroduodenal region, the site of perforation is usually readily identified. With the suction irrigator in the surgeon's right hand and a blunt grasper in the left hand, the liver edge is carefully lifted off the duodenum and pylorus. Gastric and duodenal contents are suctioned out. It is important to identify all the edges of the perforation. Ulcers in atypical locations may require additional mobilization (e.g. posterior gastric or duodenal perforation). Conversion to open laparotomy is done if the ulcer cannot be adequately exposed laparoscopically.

Primary Repair

- Three interrupted sutures are placed in a transverse manner, 2-0 or 3-0 braided sutures are used. These are placed 5–10 mm from the edges of the perforation and tied sequentially keeping the tails long. Tying these sutures requires utmost care as too tight may tear through the inflamed tissues but too loose will not close the perforation. After the perforation is closed it is covered with a tongue of healthy omentum and secured using the tails of the previously placed sutures. [29, 31–33].

Graham patch repair

- This is our preference for most small perforations. This avoids the possibility of tearing through the inflamed duodenum that can occur with primary repair. In pure omental patch repair, the interrupted sutures are placed in a transverse manner and then tied over a healthy longitudinal piece of greater omentum without first closing the perforation [24, 25, 29, 34–36]. (Fig. 8.2). A large wad of omentum is required to ensure adequate coverage. We place the uppermost suture first to ensure that the perforation will be well covered. We use different coloured sutures (neurolon (black) and vicryl (purple)) to avoid confusion when tying the omentum down.
- In order to obtain a suitable amount of mobile omentum, it may be necessary to divide the omentum vertically up to the transverse colon [30].
- In cases where the omentum cannot be used to buttress or patch the perforation, the falciform ligament can be taken down and used as a patch [24, 25, 37, 38]. Costalat et al. described using the round hepatic ligament to patch the perforation [39].

To test the integrity of the closure, saline is instilled over the repair and air is gently insufflated through the NG tube,

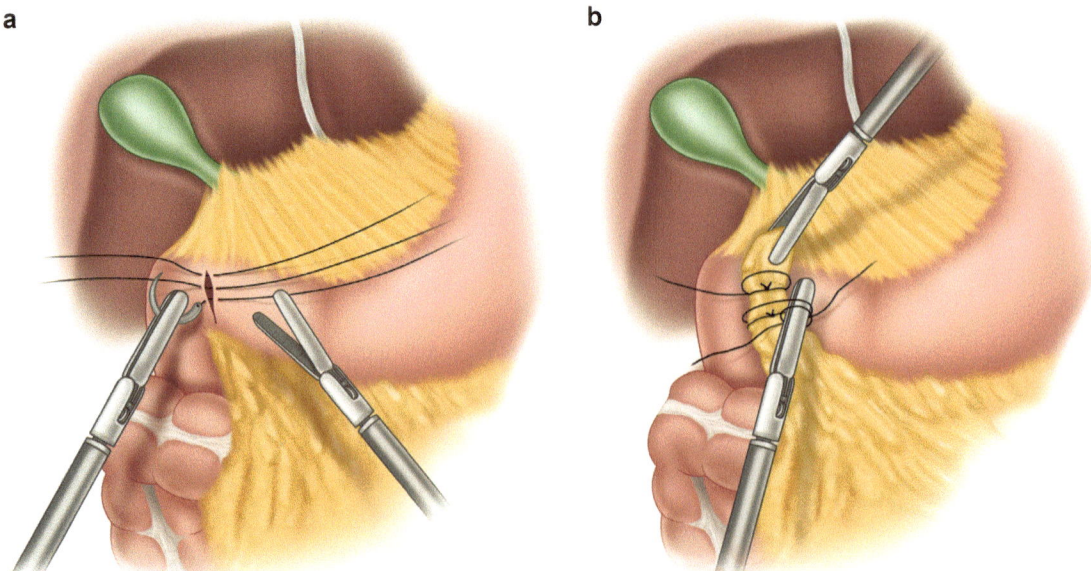

Fig. 8.2 In preparation for omental patch, three interrupted sutures are placed to traverse the ulcer perforation (**a**) [27]. The tails are left long to be tied over a healthy wad of omentum (**b**)

while the surgeon pushes down to compress the duodenum distal to the perforation to look for any air bubbles.

After the repair, extensive irrigation of the peritoneal cavity is an important step. Most authors recommend 6–10 litres of irrigation using warm normal saline [26, 34, 35, 40–43].

The final decision is whether drainage is required or not. Although we usually leave a small closed suction drain near the perforation site, this may not be necessary. In one prospective controlled study, the use of a drain did not improve post-operative pyrexia, return of bowel function or length of hospital stay and was not effective in preventing post-operative collections [44].

Conversion The conversion rate varies widely, from 0 to 60% in some studies [24, 35, 45, 46]. The most common reason to convert to open surgery is failure to identify the perforation, accounting for 31–100%, followed by large ulcer size, accounting for 20–61% [22, 24, 32, 34, 35, 45, 46]. Other reasons include patient's intolerance to pneumoperitoneum, associated bleeding from the ulcer and posterior duodenal ulcer perforation.

Post-operative Care

Post-operative care and recovery depends on the patient's physiological status and associated comorbidities. Young patients, who present early and get treated in a timely fashion, normally will have faster recovery, but older patients, who present late and have multiple associated comorbidities, might require post-operative intensive care monitoring and make a slow recovery.

The implementation of a multidisciplinary perioperative protocol to detect and treat sepsis early and standardize IV antibiotics, nutrition and fluid management [47] reduced 30-day mortality to 17% from 27% prior to the protocol.

Antibiotic Therapy Antibiotic therapy should be continued post-operatively for 2–5 days if blood cultures are negative or until fever subsides [24, 48]. Oral antibiotics are then continued as part of *Helicobacter pylori* eradication.

Nasogastric Tube and Feeding The nasogastric tube is removed when gastrointestinal function returns [24, 29, 49]. Oral feeding is then introduced and advanced as tolerated by the patient.

Eradication of *Helicobacter pylori* A meta-analysis that included five randomized control trials showed that *H. pylori* eradication significantly reduced ulcer recurrence at 8 weeks and 1 year after surgery [3, 50]. Triple therapy with proton pump inhibitor, clarithromycin and amoxicillin is recommended to continue for 14 days [51].

Follow-Up For gastric ulcers, endoscopic follow-up is performed 6 weeks after surgery to rule out the possibility of cancer [3, 49, 52]. The same is not recommended for duodenal ulcer due to the low incidence of duodenal cancer. However, eradication of *H. pylori* should be confirmed.

Complications

Leak and Infections The reported leak rate after laparoscopic repair of perforated peptic ulcer is 5–16% [21, 22, 25, 29, 45, 49]. A contained leak can usually be treated with drainage, but a persistent or uncontrolled leak requires reoperating to have source control.

Post-operative intra-abdominal abscess formation occurs in up to 9% and is treated with intravenous antibiotics and percutaneous drainage [6, 24, 25, 29, 49].

Other Complications These include superficial surgical site infection, bleeding, pneumonia, deep venous thrombosis and pulmonary embolism, prolonged ileus and gastrocutaneous or enterocutaneous fistula.

Take-Home Messages

Perforated peptic ulcer disease is a lethal disease if not treated early

Laparoscopic repair is feasible in most patients

Associated bleeding and hemodynamic instability are contraindications to laparoscopic repair

Primary closure and omentopexy or Graham patch repair can be performed

Early antibiotic therapy, irrigation and *H. pylori* eradication are essential components of therapy

---

Key References

1. Muller MK, et al. Perforated peptic ulcer repair: factors predicting conversion in laparoscopy and postoperative septic complications. World J Surg. 2016;40(9):2186–93.
2. Stewart B, et al. Global disease burden of conditions requiring emergency surgery. Br J Surg. 2014;101(1):e9–22.
3. Soreide K, et al. Perforated peptic ulcer. Lancet. 2015;386(10000):1288–98.
4. Bertleff MJ, Lange JF. Laparoscopic correction of perforated peptic ulcer: first choice? A review of literature. Surg Endosc. 2010;24(6):1231–9.
5. Wang AY, Peura DA. The prevalence and incidence of Helicobacter pylori-associated peptic ulcer disease and upper gastrointestinal bleeding throughout the world. Gastrointest Endosc Clin N Am. 2011;21(4):613–35.
6. Lau JY, et al. Systematic review of the epidemiology of complicated peptic ulcer disease: incidence, recurrence, risk factors and mortality. Digestion. 2011;84(2):102–13.
7. Wang YR, Richter JE, Dempsey DT. Trends and outcomes of hospitalizations for peptic ulcer disease in the United States, 1993 to 2006. Ann Surg. 2010;251(1):51–8.
8. Thorsen K, Soreide JA, Soreide K. What is the best predictor of mortality in perforated peptic ulcer disease? A population-based, multivariable regression analysis including three clinical scoring systems. J Gastrointest Surg. 2014;18(7):1261–8.
9. Salama NR, Hartung ML, Muller A. Life in the human stomach: persistence strategies of the bacterial pathogen Helicobacter pylori. Nat Rev Microbiol. 2013;11(6):385–99.
10. Svanes C, et al. Smoking and ulcer perforation. Gut. 1997;41(2):177–80.
11. Cid T. Pathogenesis of Helicobacter pylori infection. Helicobacter. 2013;18(Suppl 1):12–7. doi:10.1111/hel.12076.
12. Dakubo JC, Naaeder SB, Clegg-Lamptey JN. Gastro-duodenal peptic ulcer perforation. East Afr Med J. 2009;86(3):100–9.
13. Soreide K, Thorsen K, Soreide JA. Predicting outcomes in patients with perforated gastroduodenal ulcers: artificial neural network modelling indicates a highly complex disease. Eur J Trauma Emerg Surg. 2015;41(1):91–8.
14. Hirschowitz BI, Simmons J, Mohnen J. Clinical outcome using lansoprazole in acid hypersecretors with and without Zollinger-Ellison syndrome: a 13-year prospective study. Clin Gastroenterol Hepatol. 2005;3(1):39–48.
15. Kumar A, et al. The etiology of pneumoperitoneum in the 21st century. J Trauma Acute Care Surg. 2012;73(3):542–8.
16. Thorsen K, et al. Trends in diagnosis and surgical management of patients with perforated peptic ulcer. J Gastrointest Surg. 2011;15(8):1329–35.
17. Ghekiere O, et al. Value of computed tomography in the diagnosis of the cause of nontraumatic gastrointestinal tract perforation. J Comput Assist Tomogr. 2007;31(2):169–76.
18. Furukawa A, et al. Gastrointestinal tract perforation: CT diagnosis of presence, site, and cause. Abdom Imaging. 2005;30(5):524–34.
19. Taylor H. Perforated peptic ulcer; treated without operation. Lancet. 1946;2(6422):441–4.
20. Crofts TJ, et al. A randomized trial of nonoperative treatment for perforated peptic ulcer. N Engl J Med. 1989;320(15):970–3.
21. Sanabria A, Villegas MI, Morales Uribe CH. Laparoscopic repair for perforated peptic ulcer disease. Cochrane Database Syst Rev. 2013;2:CD004778.
22. Siu WT, et al. Laparoscopic repair for perforated peptic ulcer: a randomized controlled trial. Ann Surg. 2002;235(3):313–9.
23. Byrge N, et al. Laparoscopic versus open repair of perforated gastroduodenal ulcer: a National Surgical Quality Improvement Program analysis. Am J Surg. 2013;206(6):957–62. discussion 962-3
24. Lunevicius R, Morkevicius M. Management strategies, early results, benefits, and risk factors of laparoscopic repair of perforated peptic ulcer. World J Surg. 2005;29(10):1299–310.
25. Lunevicius R, Morkevicius M. Systematic review comparing laparoscopic and open repair for perforated peptic ulcer. Br J Surg. 2005;92(10):1195–207.
26. Lagoo SA, Pappas TN. Laparoscopic repair for perforated peptic ulcer. Ann Surg. 2002;235(3):320–1.
27. Lagoo S, McMahon RL, kakihara M, Pappas T, Eubanks S. The sixth decision regarding perforated duodenal ulcer. JSLS. 2002;6(4):359–68.
28. Pappas TN. Laparoscopic repair of perforated ulcer and Vagotomy. In: Pappas TN, Chekan EG, Eubanks S, editors. Atlas of laparoscopic surgery. Philadelphia: McGraw-Hill Professional Publishing; 1999.
29. Lunca Y. Laparoscopic repair of perforated peptic ulcer. Jurnalul de Chirurgie. 2007;3(2):1584–9341.
30. Mancini GJ, Mancini ML. Peptic ulcer surgery. In: Vernon AH, Ashley SW, editors. Atlas of minimally invasive surgical techniques. St Louis: Elsevier Saunders; 2012.
31. Walsh CJ, Khoo DE, Motson RW. Laparoscopic repair of perforated peptic ulcer. Br J Surg. 1993;80(1):127.
32. Michelet I, Agresta F. Perforated peptic ulcer: laparoscopic approach. Eur J Surg. 2000;166(5):405–8.

33. Nathanson LK, Easter DW, Cuschieri A. Laparoscopic repair/peritoneal toilet of perforated duodenal ulcer. Surg Endosc. 1990;4(4):232–3.

34. So JB, et al. Comparison between laparoscopic and conventional omental patch repair for perforated duodenal ulcer. Surg Endosc. 1996;10(11):1060–3.

35. Khoursheed M, et al. Laparoscopic closure of perforated duodenal ulcer. Surg Endosc. 2000;14(1):56–8.

36. Robertson GS, Wemyss-Holden SA, Maddern GJ. Laparoscopic repair of perforated peptic ulcers. The role of laparoscopy in generalised peritonitis. Ann R Coll Surg Engl. 2000;82(1):6–10.

37. Boshnaq TA, Martini I, Doughan S. Utilisation of the falciform ligament pedicle flap as an alternative approach for the repair of a perforated gastric ulcer. BMJ Case Rep. 2016;10 doi:10.1136/bcr-2015-213025.

38. Munro WS, Bajwa F, Menzies D. Laparoscopic repair of perforated duodenal ulcers with a falciform ligament patch. Ann R Coll Surg Engl. 1996;78(4):390–1.

39. Costalat G, Alquier Y. Combined laparoscopic and endoscopic treatment of perforated gastroduodenal ulcer using the ligamentum teres hepatis (LTH). Surg Endosc. 1995;9(6):677–9. discussion 680.

40. Lunevicius R, Morkevicius M. Comparison of laparoscopic versus open repair for perforated duodenal ulcers. Surg Endosc. 2005;19(12):1565–71.

41. Halkic N, Pescatore P, Gillet M. Laparoscopic-endoscopic management of perforated pyloroduodenal ulcer. Endoscopy. 1999;31(9):S64–5.

42. Matsuda M, et al. Laparoscopic omental patch repair for perforated peptic ulcer. Ann Surg. 1995;221(3):236–40.

43. Seelig MH, et al. Comparison between open and laparoscopic technique in the management of perforated gastroduodenal ulcers. J Clin Gastroenterol. 2003;37(3):226–9.

44. Pai D, et al. Role of abdominal drains in perforated duodenal ulcer patients: a prospective controlled study. Aust N Z J Surg. 1999;69(3):210–3.

45. Lee FY, et al. Predicting mortality and morbidity of patients operated on for perforated peptic ulcers. Arch Surg. 2001;136(1):90–4.

46. Thompson AR, et al. Laparoscopic plication of perforated ulcer: results of a selective approach. South Med J. 1995;88(2):185–9.

47. Moller MH, et al. Preoperative prognostic factors for mortality in peptic ulcer perforation: a systematic review. Scand J Gastroenterol. 2010;45(7–8):785–805.

48. Urbano D, et al. Alternative laparoscopic management of perforated peptic ulcers. Surg Endosc. 1994;8(10):1208–11.

49. Abd Ellatif ME, et al. Laparoscopic repair of perforated peptic ulcer: patch versus simple closure. Int J Surg. 2013;11(9):948–51.

50. Wong CS, et al. Eradication of Helicobacter pylori for prevention of ulcer recurrence after simple closure of perforated peptic ulcer: a meta-analysis of randomized controlled trials. J Surg Res. 2013;182(2):219–26.

51. Yuan Y, et al. Optimum duration of regimens for Helicobacter pylori eradication. Cochrane Database Syst Rev. 2013;12:CD008337.

52. Kumar P, Khan HM, Hasanrabba S. Treatment of perforated giant gastric ulcer in an emergency setting. World J Gastrointest Surg. 2014;6(1):5–8.

Suggested Reading

Bertleff MJ, Lange JF. Laparoscopic correction of perforated peptic ulcer: first choice? A review of literature. Surg Endosc. 2010;24:1231–9.

Lunevicius R, Morkevicius M. Management strategies, early results, benefits, and risk factors of laparoscopic repair of perforated peptic ulcer. World J Surg. 2005;29:1299–310. doi:10.1007/s00268-005-7705-4.

Muller M, Wrann S, Widmer J, Klasen J, Weber M, Hahnloser D. Perforated peptic ulcer repair: factors predicting conversion in laparoscopy and postoperative septic complications. World J Surg. 2016;40(9):2186–93.

Sanabria A, Villegas MI, Morales Uribe CH. Laparoscopic repair for perforated peptic ulcer disease. Cochrane Database Syst Rev. 2013;2:CD004778.

Søreide K, Thorsen K, Harrison EM, Bingener J, Møller MH, Ohene-Yeboah M, Søreide JA. Perforated peptic ulcer. Lancet. 2015;386:1288–98.

Minimally Invasive Strategies
for the Treatment of Necrotizing
Infected Pancreatitis: Video-Assisted
Retroperitoneal Debridement (VARD)

9

Jacques Mather and Jose J. Diaz

Introduction

The first descriptions of pancreatitis can be traced back to the Dutch anatomist and surgeon Nicolaes Tulp in the mid-seventeenth century. In the 350 years since, much progress has been made in medicine and in our understanding of the pathophysiology of disease. Yet despite these advances, pancreatitis remains a disease with outcomes difficult to predict and treatments often left in the realm of "supportive care," thus consistent with Tulp's description of the pancreas as "Pandora's box." Nonetheless, in the last few decades, tremendous strides have been made in the understanding and treatment of acute pancreatitis.

At its most basic level, pancreatitis describes a pathologic inflammatory state of the pancreas or the peripancreatic tissue. It is commonly associated with gallstone disease or alcohol use and can have a wide spectrum of physiologic manifestations. Patients are generally very dehydrated from an inflammatory state that leads to relative intravascular volume depletion which may be further exacerbated by invariable nausea and vomiting. Treatment begins with fluid resuscitation for all patients. Those who present in a more advanced state of the disease process may require large volumes of intravenous fluid, ventilator support, and monitoring in an ICU setting.

In cases of necrotizing or infected pancreatitis, activated pancreatic enzymes cause autodigestion of the pancreatic tissue and lead to the development of peripancreatic fluid collections and cell death. These collections can then coalesce to form pseudocysts or walled-off pancreatic necrosis (WOPN).

J. Mather (✉)
Program in Trauma, R Adams Cowley Shock Trauma Center, University of Maryland Medical Center, Baltimore, MD, USA
e-mail: jpmather@gmail.com

J.J. Diaz
Chief Division of Acute Care Surgery, Acute Care Surgery Fellowship, Program in Trauma, R Adams Cowley Shock Trauma Center, University of Maryland Medical Center, Baltimore, MD, USA

Devitalized tissue with an area of WOPN can be a nidus for infection and allow for the development of infected necrosis.

Although pancreatitis is a mild illness in the majority of cases, severe acute pancreatitis continues to have a high morbidity and mortality rate. In 2009, acute pancreatitis was the most commonly diagnosed gastrointestinal disorder accounting for approximately 270,000 hospital admissions. Moreover, its financial effect on the healthcare system is estimated at almost three billion dollars per year in inpatient hospital costs [1]. Fortunately, as most cases are mild, mortality hovers around 1%. Mortality, however, increases to almost 30% if either organ failure or infected pancreatic necrosis is present. If both are present together, mortality approaches 43% [2].

Defining Acute Pancreatitis

In 1992, the Atlanta Symposium sought to provide a classification system for acute pancreatitis that would allow clinicians to standardize their approach to management [3]. With advances in technology and understanding of acute pancreatitis, there became a need to update this classification system, and in 2012, the revised Atlanta Classification was produced. It developed new criteria for diagnosing acute pancreatitis, defining morphology, and classifying severity [4]. Three forms of acute pancreatitis are described: mild, moderately severe, and severe. In mild acute pancreatitis, patients have no evidence of organ failure or any local or systemic complications. Pain often resolves rapidly with bowel rest and hydration, and they can often be discharged early. Patients with moderately severe acute pancreatitis will have evidence of *transient* organ failure (persisting for less than 48 h), or they will have local or systemic complications in the absence of organ failure. While many patients will recover rapidly, some may require prolonged care before full recovery. Finally, in patients with severe acute pancreatitis, organ failure persists for greater than 48 h. Mortality in this group is much higher than those in either the mild or the moderately severe group [5].

In order to diagnose acute pancreatitis, two of the three following criteria must be met: the patient must have (1) abdominal pain that is consistent with acute pancreatitis, (2) serum lipase or amylase activity that is at least three times greater than the upper limit of normal, or (3) contrast-enhanced computed tomography (CECT) with characteristic findings of acute pancreatitis. Acute pancreatitis can then be classified into either an "interstitial edematous" form or a "necrotizing" form. This classification is not mutually exclusive, and both forms most likely fall along the same spectrum of the disease process. The majority of patients fall into interstitial edematous category. However, approximately 5–10% will eventually develop pancreatic or peripancreatic necrosis (or both) [5]. It is important to note that early CECT may underestimate necrosis, as it likely requires several days to fully evolve [4]. Thus, delaying CECT, if a patient meets the other two criteria, is appropriate.

Infection of necrotic pancreatic or peripancreatic tissue (Fig. 9.1) is a highly morbid yet poorly predictable complication. There does not appear to be a correlation between amount of necrotic tissue and likelihood of infection, and it is an extremely unusual diagnosis in the first week of symptoms. Nonetheless, recognition of infection is vital as it alters the treatment strategy, requires antibiotics, and may ultimately require intervention.

Interventions

The decision to proceed with interventions in patients with necrotizing pancreatitis revolves around the evidence for infection, whether based on a positive Gram stain or culture from an FNA, the presence of gas on CT-imaging, or a persistent sepsis in the context of known acute pancreatitis.

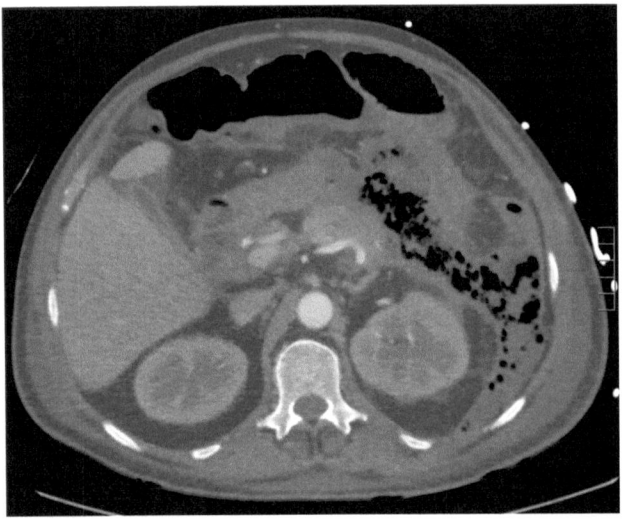

Fig. 9.1 Large peripancreatic collection of fluid gas consistent with infected pancreatic necrosis

Management still begins with conventional methods, including intravenous fluid administration and symptomatic treatment. For these patients, broad-spectrum antibiotics are also started [6]. Early surgical intervention has been proven time and time again to be associated with unacceptably high mortality rates [7] and should be avoided. Thus, aggressive ICU management in the first 4 weeks of symptoms will hopefully avoid surgical intervention within this early window. This period of time allows the collections to mature and "wall off," thereby improving the surgical conditions. Percutaneous drainage during this timeframe can help to "bridge" the patient to an eventual intervention or may prove to be the only treatment necessary. The goal of intervention in infected necrotizing pancreatitis is the same as that for any infection: source control. Attempts in the past to aggressively manage this disease process via large open incisions with complete removal of not only the infection but also all necrotic pancreatic tissue resulted in significant morbidity and mortality. Evidence is now suggesting that clearing of the infection alone without aggressive removal of all necrotic tissue is likely associated with better outcomes including reduced morbidity, mortality, length of hospital stay, and in-hospital costs [8, 9].

Maximally Invasive Methods

For decades, an open surgical approach was considered the optimal strategy for removing all of the infected and necrotic pancreatic or peripancreatic tissue. Beger and colleagues [10] first described this intervention in 1988, which included either a midline laparotomy incision or a bilateral subcostal incision, entrance into the lesser sac for debridement, and postoperative local lavage of the pancreatic bed. A year later, in 1989, Fagniez described a translumbar retroperitoneal approach [11], which involved a 20-cm left lateral incision just anterior to the 12th rib and provided direct retroperitoneal access, avoiding the peritoneal cavity yet allowing a great deal of access to the retroperitoneum. Complications, however, were not uncommon and included hemorrhage; colonic, small bowel, and pancreatic fistulae; and bowel ischemia [12]. "Open" approaches are, therefore, highly morbid and expose an already sick patient to an extensive operation with a number of potential complications. In this minimally invasive era, the primary indications for open necrosectomy include inability to reach the collection minimally invasively (e.g., a remaining central collection), persistent hemodynamic instability despite resuscitation, and intra-abdominal collections.

Minimally Invasive Methods

Given the morbidity of open surgery, a number of operative strategies have been proposed as alternatives. These strategies, generally considered "minimally invasive," accomplish debridement of necrotic tissue via percutaneous, endoscopic, or laparoscopic routes. An array of techniques has been described to provide direct access and direct visualization of the necrotic cavity, including the use of transgastric or transduodenal endoscopy as well as laparoscopy [8, 13, 14]. The literature also includes examples of the use of mediastinoscopes [15] and nephroscopes [16] to gain visualization and a working space in the retroperitoneum. The Dutch Acute Pancreatitis Study Group, in 2006, proposed a "step-up approach" to managing infected acute necrotizing pancreatitis [17] with the goal of beginning treatment with less invasive approaches and maximizing therapy gradually if the previous interventions failed. Management can begin with a percutaneous or endoscopic procedure to allow for minimally invasive drainage of the infected material with the initial goal of controlling sepsis, with a secondary goal of eradicating the collection. If this intervention fails, the authors recommend moving to a minimally invasive retroperitoneal necrosectomy. Only in the context of failure of these strategies or significant complications would an open necrosectomy be recommended. This study, also known as the PANTER trial, demonstrated a significant decrease in complication rates between an open necrosectomy group and a "step-up" group (40% vs 12%), although mortality rates were similar [9]. Advantages of a minimally invasive approach when compared with open surgery include shorter ICU stays and faster recovery, decreased multisystem organ failure, a lessened inflammatory response, and lesser chance of perpetuating bacteremia. The retroperitoneal approach also reduces potential violation of the peritoneal cavity and decreases the chance of hollow viscus injury. Multiple case series involving minimally invasive approaches have shown lower mortality rates; however, none compare these techniques with open necrosectomy [18–20].

Percutaneous Drainage

The first step in the "step-up" approach is percutaneous image-guided catheter drainage of pancreatic and/or peripancreatic collections. Freeny et al. in 1998 was the first group to study percutaneous drainage of infected pancreatic necrosis [21]. They evaluated 34 patients and had a 47% success rate, defined as complete resolution of the collection, with a 12% mortality rate. Their technique required multiple catheters and frequent catheter upsizing. When this technique is used alone, it frequently requires conversion to more invasive procedures. Loculated collections and solidified necrotic material are, in particular, not easily amenable to percutaneous drainage; thus it is also often utilized as a temporizing method during the "early window" to delay surgical intervention. There are, however, a number of potential ben-

efits: it can be done under minimal anesthetic requirements, most collections are accessible for drainage under radiological guidance, it can be performed in the early stages of pancreatitis, complications are few, and morbidity and mortality from the procedure are low. Perhaps most importantly, if percutaneous drainage is successful, the patient will likely require no further interventions (Figs. 9.2 and 9.3).

Laparoscopy/Video-Assisted Retroperitoneal Debridement (VARD) in Acute Necrotizing Pancreatitis

Greater than half of the time, however, percutaneous drainage is not sufficient for resolution [8]. Of the various additional techniques, video-assisted retroperitoneal debridement (VARD) has been garnering a great deal of enthusiasm (Table 9.1). Horvath et al. in 2001, using the term "laparoscopic-assisted percutaneous debridement," first described this technique and its use on six patients [22, 25]. In 2007, Van Santvoort and the Dutch Acute Pancreatitis Study Group also published their technique with some minor differences [23, 26]. VARD effectively combines percutaneous drainage with a minimally invasive retroperitoneal approach and laparoscopic guidance. With a percutaneous drain in place within the pancreatic collection, the patient is taken to the operating room, and, using the drain as a road map, a space is opened within the retroperitoneum that allows placement of a finger, a Yankauer, a laparoscopic camera, and a grasper all of which can be used to carefully remove and debride infected tissue (See Figs. 9.4, 9.5, 9.6, 9.7 and 9.8). The operative steps are shown in Fig. 9.9 [18, 25, 26].

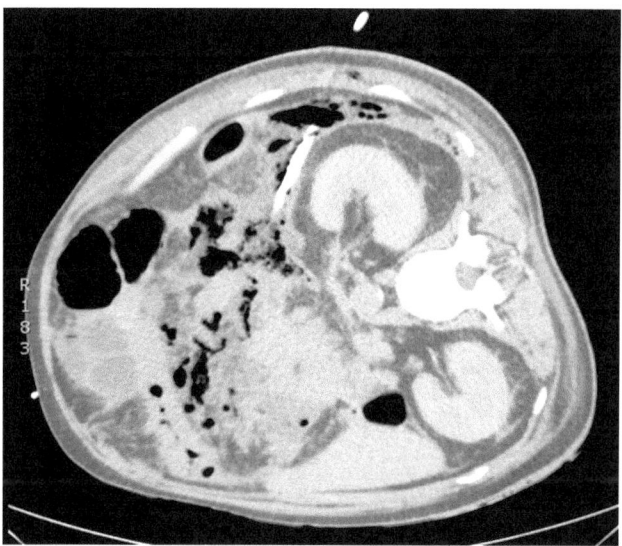

Fig. 9.2 Percutaneous drain placed into pancreatic collection

Table 9.1 Outcomes of previous VARD studies

Author (year)	Study type	Total patients[a]	VARD patients	Time to intervention, Avg. days [range]	Complications, n (%)[b]	Conversion to open, n (%)	Mortality (%)	Perc. drain only success	Overall minimally invasive success rate, %
Horvath (2001) [22]	Retrospective	6	6	40.5 [27–77]	2 (33)	2 (33)	0	0	66
Van Santvoort (2007) [23]	Retrospective, case matched	15	15	41 [15–149]	6 (40)	4 (27)	1 (7)	NR	73
Horvath (2010) [24]	Multicenter, prospective cohort	34	25	49 [0–209]	10 (29)	10 (40)	1 (6)	9 (26)	71
Van Santvoort (2010) [9]	Multicenter, randomly controlled, prospective	43	24	30 [11–71]	23 (53)	1 (4)	8 (19)	15 (35)	60
García-Ureña (2013) [18]	Case series	7	7	30 [12–76]	3 (43)	0	0	NR	100
Šileikis (2013) [20]	Retrospective	13	13	25.7 [14–37]	2 (15)	2 (15)	0	NR	85
Perumal (2013) [19]	Retrospective	39	26	47 [12–82]	11 (42)	1 (4)	2 (8)	13 (33)	88

NR not reported

[a]Includes only patients treated with minimally invasive methods

[b]Complications include both intraoperative and postoperative, such as bleeding, development of fistulae, bowel ischemia, etc. Not included are additional VARD or percutaneous procedures for further debridement.

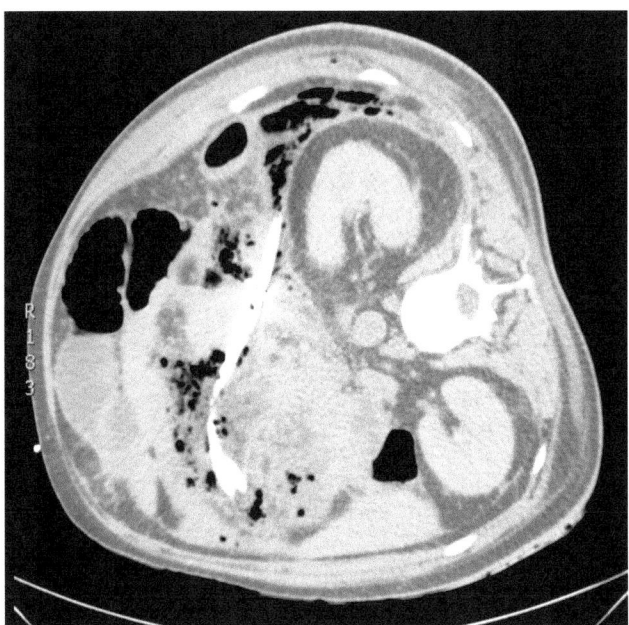

Fig. 9.3 Percutaneous drain is large bore and extends throughout the collection

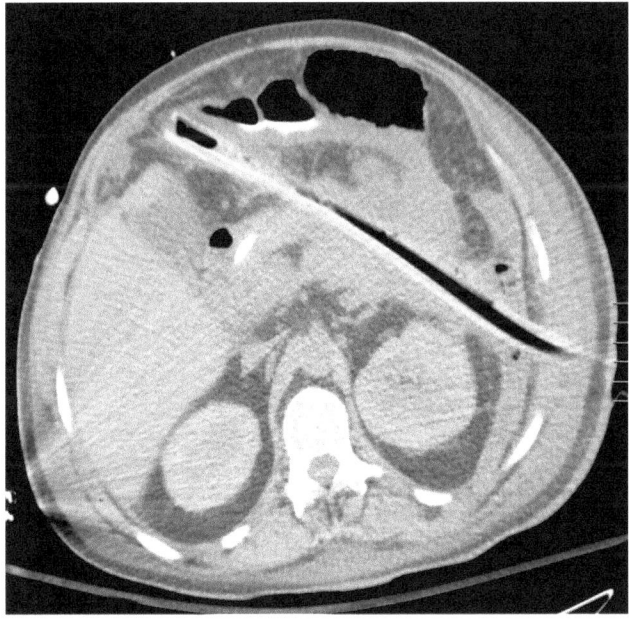

Fig. 9.4 Large bore drain placed at completion of VARD

In the initial series of six patients, Horvath and colleagues were able to avoid open necrosectomy in four of the patients, and all of the patients survived. The "step-up" approach was published in the New England Journal of Medicine almost a decade later, which randomized patients to either an open necrosectomy or a minimally invasive step-up approach [9]. Of those treated minimally invasively, 35% required percutaneous drainage alone. Over 90% of the remaining patients underwent VARD. Compared with open necrosectomy,

patients in the minimally invasive group were significantly less likely to have a major complication, in particular multi-system organ failure or other major systemic complications. These patients were also significantly less likely to be admitted to the ICU following their intervention. However, there were no differences between the groups in development of enteric or pancreatic fistulae and in intra-abdominal bleeding requiring intervention nor were there differences in overall mortality. Long-term outcomes favored the minimally invasive group as they experienced less instances of new-onset diabetes, requirements for pancreatic enzyme replacement, and incisional hernias.

Safety and efficacy of VARD have since been demonstrated [24], and, similar to percutaneous drainage, some patients will require more than one VARD procedure to adequately control the infection. The majority of these patients also go on to cure rather than requiring conversion to open necrosectomy. Unfortunately, to date, no studies have been published comparing VARD with other minimally invasive techniques nor as of yet are there any new studies comparing VARD with open necrosectomy.

Further modifications to the VARD technique have also been published. Zhao et al. describe a technique of "retro-peritoneoscopic anatomical necrosectomy (REAN)" which involves access to the retroperitoneum without the requirement of a percutaneous catheter for guidance [27]. They suggest that this approach allows for complete necrotic tissue debridement and easier drainage. Sileikis et al. describe the use of three separate ports [28], and Wronski and colleagues utilize a single-incision laparoscopic surgery (SILS) port for access and debridement [29]. Figure 9.10 provides an algorithm for management of acute pancreatitis including indications for VARD.

Complications

Given the tenuous nature of patients with severe necrotizing pancreatitis and the real estate surrounding the debridement area, complications from this procedure are often unavoidable and include SIRS/sepsis, hemorrhage, enteric and pancreatic fistulae, and hollow viscus and solid organ injury [5, 30, 31]. Hemorrhage is a particularly daunting complication, and immediate management may require laparotomy, interventional radiology, or even, as reported by the group at the R Adams Cowley Shock Trauma Center, placement of a resuscitative balloon occlusion of the aorta (REBOA) for control [32]. Early hemorrhage may accompany an overly aggressive debridement, and attempted management via open surgical approaches often results in mortality. These situations may best be served with packing or even balloon tamponade. If the source is arterial, emergency angiography should be considered. In the case of venous bleeding, pack-

Fig. 9.5 VARD operative
steps

VARD operative steps
1. With a percutaneous drain in place, a post-drain CT scan is obtained to determine the three-dimensional location of the catheter.
2. The patient is then taken the operating room and placed in supine position with the left side bumped up approximately 30 to 40° to allow for direct access to the left paracolic gutter, but also rapid access for a laparotomy if necessary. If the patient has a collection along the right gutter consider positioning with the right side elevated.
3. A 5-cm subcostal incision is made anterior to posterior centering along the mid-axillary line near to or including the drain exit site.
4. Digital dissection then proceeds deeply but cautiously along the drain. The fascia is incised allowing entrance into the retroperitoneum and access to the pancreatic necrosectum; it is important to identify and avoid the colon anteriorly.
5. Initial purulent material can be carefully removed with a suction device or a pair of long forceps.
6. Necrotic material that is directly identifiable and easily mobilized can also be removed digitally.
7. Once direct visualization of the necrotic material is no longer possible a single, extra-long, blunt laparoscopic port is placed through the wound following the course of the drain; a 0° laparoscope is introduced and CO_2 is used for insufflation via the percutaneous drain up to 14 mmHg.
8. Leakage of insufflated gas can be prevented by placing wet towels in the wound and around the port.
9. Using laparoscopic graspers, further debridement can be done under direct visualization. Debride cautiously and avoid tight bands that cross through the space as these are likely blood vessels.
10. Copious irrigation in conjunction with laparoscopic graspers can be used for debridement of the necrotic pancreatic tissue. It is not necessary to remove all of the necrotic tissue; only remove tissue that is easy to mobilize.
11. Pulse irrigation to the cavity should be performed with 4-6 L of saline until output clears.
12. Create an irrigation system for post-operative management. Remove the percutaneous drain and place two large bore catheters (one at the deepest point and one superficial) into the cavity and bring them out either through a separate stab incision or through the initial incision. Penrose drains can also be used. Fascia and skin are closed.
13. Post-operative continuous lavage via the deep catheter is commenced at 10L/day for 5 days. Effluent is collected through the superficial drain.
14. Serial CT scans should be done every 5-7 days to evaluate for improvement in the pancreatic collection.

ing of the wound and correction of coagulopathy should be the goal. Delayed hemorrhage is often arterial in nature and can present as a "herald" bleed per the retroperitoneal drains or via the GI tract. Rapid assessment, high clinical suspicion, rapid CT angiogram, or engagement of emergency angiographic procedures can be lifesaving.

Enteric fistulas, especially gastric or proximal small bowel, may present in an insidious manner and may accompany improvements in the patient's condition as these can mimic the similar endoscopic drainage procedures. Colonic fistulae, however, may lead to persistent sepsis and ultimately require either resection of fistulous segment or proximal diversion if they fail to close spontaneously. Pancreatic fistulae are managed principally by catheter-based drainage.

Early ERCP in this patient population especially with persistent collections can potentially be detrimental and lead to the introduction of infection. Therefore, current recommendations are to maintain prolonged drainage to allow maturation of the tract with interval removal of the drain [5]. This will often lead to spontaneous closure of the fistula. If resolution of the collection and the septic picture have been achieved, ERCP may be appropriate with introduction of a pancreatic ductal stent to attempt fistula closure.

Finally, all of these approaches lend themselves to hollow viscus and solid organ injury. Particularly at risk are the stomach, left colon, and spleen. But injuries to the left kidney, mesenteric defunctionalization, and major vascular injuries have all been reported.

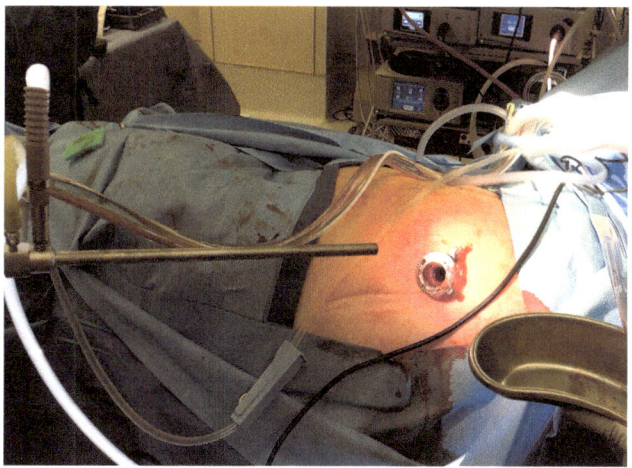

Fig. 9.6 Single laparoscopic port placed via a retroperitoneal incision. Incision closed around port to help maintain insufflation

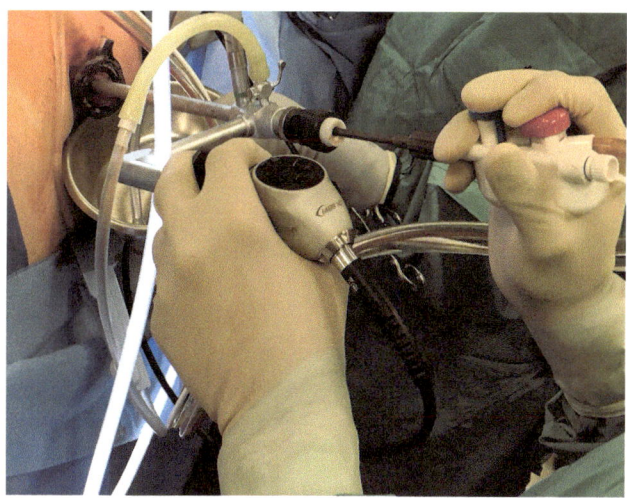

Fig. 9.7 Irrigation of the retroperitoneal cavity through single right-angled laparoscope with a working port

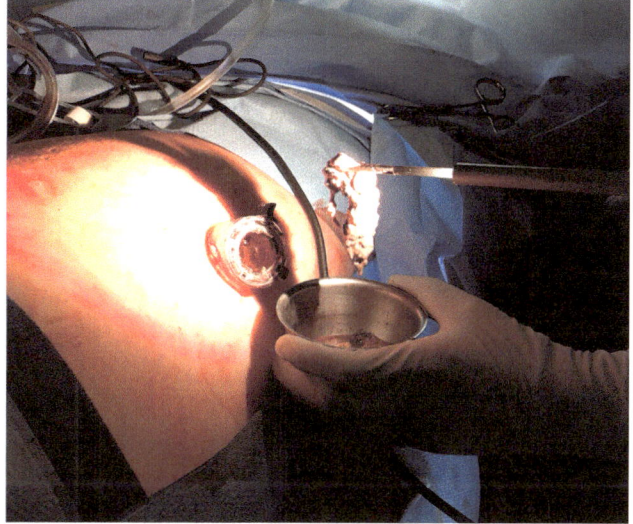

Fig. 9.8 Necrotic peripancreatic tissue being removed with a laparoscopic grasper

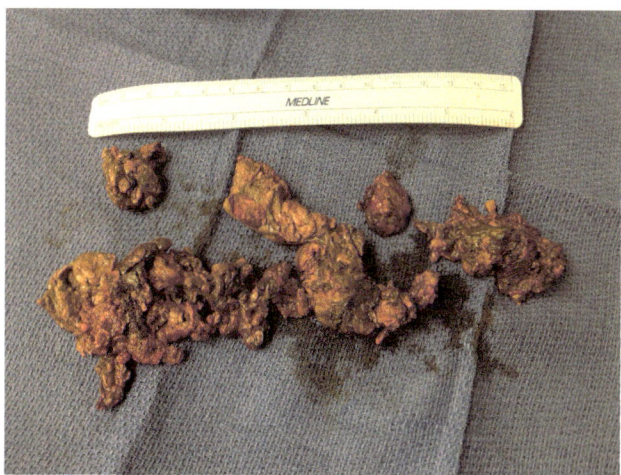

Fig. 9.9 Examples of necrotic tissue removed during a VARD procedure

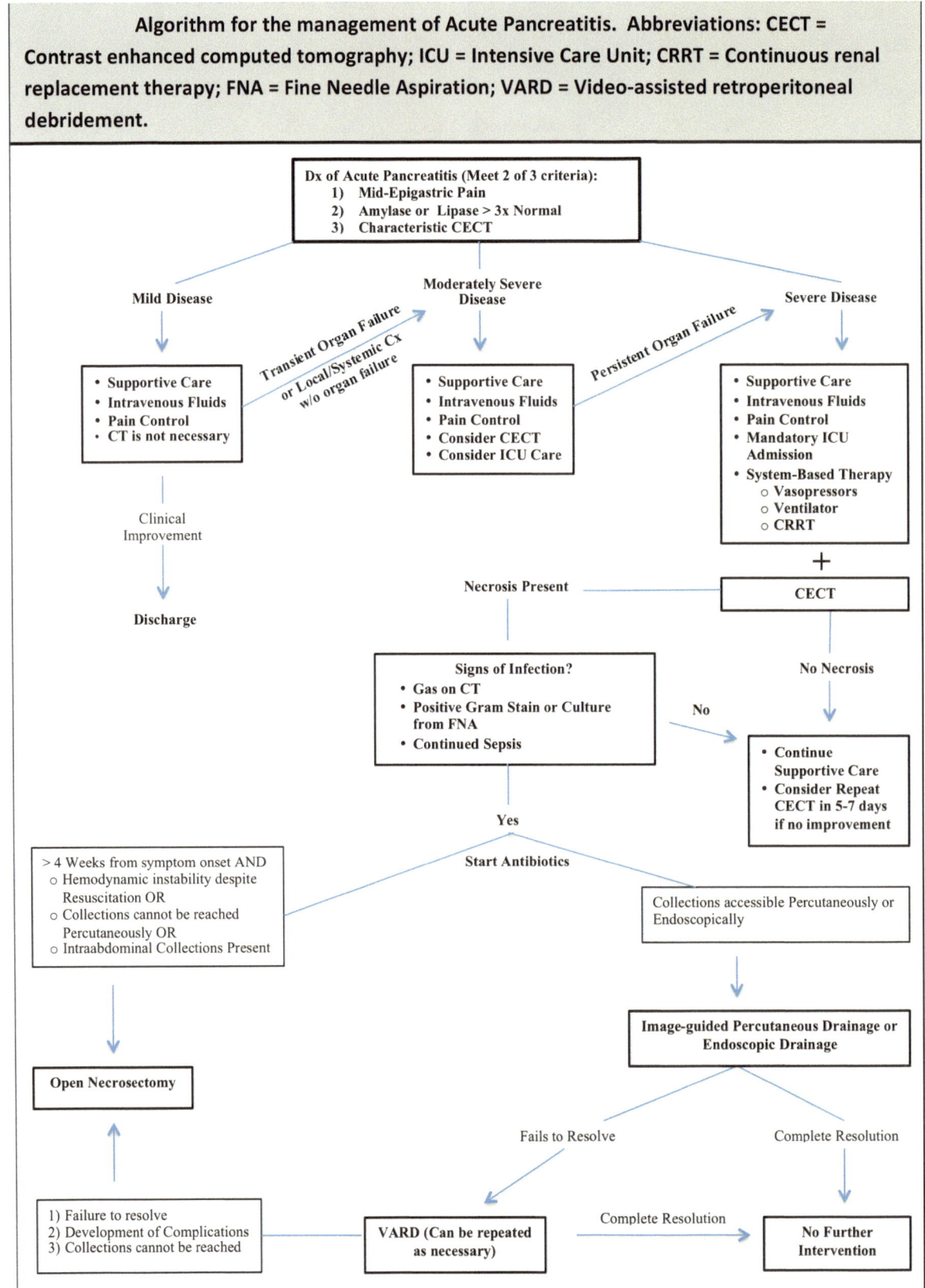

Fig. 9.10 Algorithm for the management of acute pancreatitis. Abbreviations: *CECT* contrast-enhanced computed tomography, *ICU* intensive care unit, *CRRT* continuous renal replacement therapy, *FNA* fine needle aspiration, *VARD* video-assisted retroperitoneal debridement

Take-Home Messages

1. Surgical management of acute necrotizing pancreatitis should occur in a planned and staged approach. The ideal scenario is to avoid early intervention (<2 weeks) if at all possible. Current indications for early surgical interventions are abdominal compartment syndrome and bowel perforation.

2. Infected pancreatic necrosis should initially be managed with percutaneous drainage. The 2016 SCCM Surviving Sepsis Guidelines recommend percutaneous drainage as a first step in the management of the septic patient with infected pancreatic necrosis. The drain should ideally be placed in the retroperitoneum for future VARDS approach.

3. Planning for a VARDS procedure starts early in the course of the patient who develops infected pancreatic necrosis. The timing of drain placement and the course of the percutaneous drain are vitally important and require a combined effort from the surgeon and the interventional radiologist.

Key References

1. Peery AF, Dellon ES, Lund J, Crockett SD, McGowan CE, Bulsiewicz WJ, et al. Burden of gastrointestinal disease in the United States: 2012 update. Gastroenterology. 2012;143(5):1179–87. e1-3.
2. Petrov MS, Shanbhag S, Chakraborty M, Phillips AR, Windsor JA. Organ failure and infection of pancreatic necrosis as determinants of mortality in patients with acute pancreatitis. Gastroenterology. 2010;139(3):813–20.
3. Bradley EL 3rd. A clinically based classification system for acute pancreatitis. Summary of the International Symposium on Acute Pancreatitis, Atlanta, Ga, September 11 through 13, 1992. Arch Surg. 1993;128(5):586–90.
4. Banks PA, Bollen TL, Dervenis C, Gooszen HG, Johnson CD, Sarr MG, et al. Classification of acute pancreatitis–2012: revision of the Atlanta classification and definitions by international consensus. Gut. 2013;62(1):102–11.
5. Logue JA, Carter CR. Minimally invasive Necrosectomy techniques in severe acute pancreatitis: role of percutaneous Necrosectomy and video-assisted retroperitoneal debridement. Gastroenterol Res Pract. 2015;2015:693040.
6. Working Group IAPAPAAPG. IAP/APA evidence-based guidelines for the management of acute pancreatitis. Pancreatology. 2013;13(4 Suppl 2):e1–15.
7. Mier J, Leon EL, Castillo A, Robledo F, Blanco R. Early versus late necrosectomy in severe necrotizing pancreatitis. Am J Surg. 1997;173(2):71–5.
8. Wronski M, Cebulski W, Slodkowski M, Krasnodebski IW. Minimally invasive treatment of infected pancreatic necrosis. Prz Gastroenterol. 2014;9(6):317–24.
9. van Santvoort HC, Besselink MG, Bakker OJ, Hofker HS, Boermeester MA, Dejong CH, et al. A step-up approach or open necrosectomy for necrotizing pancreatitis. N Engl J Med. 2010;362(16):1491–502.
10. Beger HG, Buchler M, Bittner R, Oettinger W, Block S, Nevalainen T. Necrosectomy and postoperative local lavage in patients with necrotizing pancreatitis: results of a prospective clinical trial. World J Surg. 1988;12(2):255–62.
11. Fagniez PL, Rotman N, Kracht M. Direct retroperitoneal approach to necrosis in severe acute pancreatitis. Br J Surg. 1989;76(3):264–7.
12. Nieuwenhuijs VB, Besselink MG, van Minnen LP, Gooszen HG. Surgical management of acute necrotizing pancreatitis: a 13-year experience and a systematic review. Scand J Gastroenterol Suppl. 2003;239:111–6.
13. Gagner M. Laparoscopic treatment of acute necrotizing pancreatitis. Semin Laparosc Surg. 1996;3(1):21–8.
14. Connor S, Ghaneh P, Raraty M, Sutton R, Rosso E, Garvey CJ, et al. Minimally invasive retroperitoneal pancreatic necrosectomy. Dig Surg. 2003;20(4):270–7.
15. Gambiez LP, Denimal FA, Porte HL, Saudemont A, Chambon JP, Quandalle PA. Retroperitoneal approach and endoscopic management of peripancreatic necrosis collections. Arch Surg. 1998;133(1):66–72.
16. Carter CR, McKay CJ, Imrie CW. Percutaneous necrosectomy and sinus tract endoscopy in the management of infected pancreatic necrosis: an initial experience. Ann Surg. 2000;232(2):175–80.
17. Besselink MG, van Santvoort HC, Nieuwenhuijs VB, Boermeester MA, Bollen TL, Buskens E, et al. Minimally invasive 'step-up approach' versus maximal necrosectomy in patients with acute necrotising pancreatitis (PANTER trial): design and rationale of a randomised controlled multicenter trial [ISRCTN13975868]. BMC Surg. 2006;6:6.
18. Garcia-Urena MA, Lopez-Monclus J, Melero-Montes D, Blazquez-Hernando LA, Castellon-Pavon C, Calvo-Duran E, et al. Video-assisted laparoscopic debridement for retroperitoneal pancreatic collections: a reliable step-up approach. Am Surg. 2013;79(4):429–33.
19. Ulagendra Perumal S, Pillai SA, Perumal S, Sathyanesan J, Palaniappan R. Outcome of video-assisted translumbar retroperitoneal necrosectomy and closed lavage for severe necrotizing pancreatitis. ANZ J Surg. 2014;84(4):270–4.
20. Sileikis A, Beisa V, Beisa A, Samuilis A, Serpytis M, Strupas K. Minimally invasive retroperitoneal necrosectomy in management of acute necrotizing pancreatitis. Wideochir Inne Tech Maloinwazyjne. 2013;8(1):29–35.
21. Freeny PC, Hauptmann E, Althaus SJ, Traverso LW, Sinanan M. Percutaneous CT-guided catheter drainage of infected acute necrotizing pancreatitis: techniques and results. AJR Am J Roentgenol. 1998;170(4):969–75.
22. Horvath KD, Kao LS, Ali A, Wherry KL, Pellegrini CA, Sinanan MN. Laparoscopic assisted percutaneous drainage of infected pancreatic necrosis. Surg Endosc. 2001;15(7):677–82.
23. van Santvoort HC, Besselink MG, Bollen TL, Buskens E, van Ramshorst B, Gooszen HG, et al. Case-matched comparison of the retroperitoneal approach with laparotomy for necrotizing pancreatitis. World J Surg. 2007;31(8):1635–42.
24. Horvath K, Freeny P, Escallon J, Heagerty P, Comstock B, Glickerman DJ, et al. Safety and efficacy of video-assisted retroperitoneal debridement for infected pancreatic collections: a multicenter, prospective, single-arm phase 2 study. Arch Surg. 2010;145(9):817–25.
25. Horvath KD, Kao LS, Wherry KL, Pellegrini CA, Sinanan MN. A technique for laparoscopic-assisted percutaneous drainage of infected pancreatic necrosis and pancreatic abscess. Surg Endosc. 2001;15(10):1221–5.
26. van Santvoort HC, Besselink MG, Horvath KD, Sinanan MN, Bollen TL, van Ramshorst B, et al. Videoscopic assisted retroperitoneal debridement in infected necrotizing pancreatitis. HPB (Oxford). 2007;9(2):156–9.
27. Zhao G, Hu M, Liu R, Xu Y. Retroperitoneoscopic anatomical Necrosectomy: a modified single-stage video-assisted retroperitoneal approach for treatment of infected necrotizing pancreatitis. Surg Innov. 2015;22(4):360–5.

28. Sileikis A, Beisa V, Simutis G, Tamosiunas A, Strupas K. Three-port retroperitoneoscopic necrosectomy in management of acute necrotic pancreatitis. Medicina (Kaunas). 2010;46(3):176–9.

29. Wronski M, Cebulski W, Slodkowski M, Karkocha D, Krasnodebski IW. Retroperitoneal minimally invasive pancreatic necrosectomy using single-port access. Surg Laparosc Endosc Percutan Tech. 2012;22(1):e8–11.

30. Lim E, Sundaraamoorthy RS, Tan D, Teh HS, Tan TJ, Cheng A. Step-up approach and video assisted retroperitoneal debridement in infected necrotizing pancreatitis: a case complicated by retroperitoneal bleeding and colonic fistula. Ann Med Surg (Lond). 2015;4(3):225–9.

31. Connor S, Alexakis N, Raraty MG, Ghaneh P, Evans J, Hughes M, et al. Early and late complications after pancreatic necrosectomy. Surgery. 2005;137(5):499–505.

32. Weltz AS, Harris DG, O'Neill NA, O'Meara LB, Brenner ML, Diaz JJ. The use of resuscitative endovascular balloon occlusion of the aorta to control hemorrhagic shock during video-assisted retroperitoneal debridement or infected necrotizing pancreatitis. Int J Surg Case Rep. 2015;13:15–8.

John Hagen

Overview

Small bowel obstructions from any etiology can be managed laparoscopically. There been some controversy as to the safety of laparoscopy because of the concern that dilated small bowel could be injured either with insertion of the first port or with laparoscopic manipulation [1, 8]. The initial management will depend upon the suspected etiology of the small bowel obstruction. The usual surgical principles should be applied of nasogastric suction, intravenous fluids, and stabilization of the patient. Special attention should be made to the insertion of the first port to avoid injury to the dilated loops of the small intestine. This chapter will deal with the safe management of small bowel obstruction laparoscopically.

Patient Selection

The number of patients with small bowel obstruction that are managed laparoscopically is increasing [14]. Depending on the surgeon's skill and experience, most patients with small bowel obstruction needing surgical intervention can be considered for a laparoscopic approach as they may benefit from lower rates of complications [4, 14, 15]. However, patients that are hemodynamically unstable or those that may not be able to tolerate pneumoperitoneum because of medical conditions such as cardiac or respiratory issues may best be managed with laparotomy. If the patient has a known fused (or "frozen") abdomen from previous surgery, it may be

hazardous to attempt pneumoperitoneum, and this patient may be best managed with a laparotomy.

Definition

Small bowel obstruction is defined as a mechanical blockage of small intestine preventing normal passage of gas and small intestinal contents through to the colon. The causes include postoperative adhesions, hernias, food bolus, gallstone ileus, foreign bodies, tumors, and postoperative small bowel obstruction within a few days of surgery [2].

Laparoscopic Exploration for Small Bowel Obstruction

The position of the patient for laparoscopic small bowel obstruction is with the arms tucked at the side so that access to all four quadrants of the abdomen is possible. It is helpful to use a bean bag to prevent the patient from slipping on the table so that you can place the patient in extreme Trendelenburg or reverse Trendelenburg if necessary. Many times, there is a midline incision from previous laparotomy. One of the safest places for entry is in the left upper quadrant. A small incision is made and a Veress needle is inserted. The abdomen is insufflated with carbon dioxide to a pressure of 12–15 mm Hg. The first port is inserted under direct vision using a non-cutting trocar. Once the first port is inserted, you can determine where the other ports can be placed. If the umbilicus is free of adhesions, a port can be placed there.

If there is no midline incision, the first port can be placed using the open technique through the umbilicus. The other ports can be placed depending on the findings at the time of laparoscopy. Typically, three additional ports are used, one on the right side and two on the left. If there has been a previous laparotomy, adhesions will likely be encountered. Adhesions should be taken down with sharp dissection, and

Electronic supplementary material The online version of this chapter (doi:10.1007/978-3-319-64723-4_10) contains supplementary material, which is available to authorized users.

J. Hagen (✉)
Department of Surgery University of Toronto, Humber River Hospital, Toronto, ON, Canada
e-mail: johnhagen@bellnet.ca; jhagen@drjohnhagen.com

energy sources should be avoided to avoid inadvertent enterotomy. Gentle pressure can be applied to the distended bowel with the graspers, but manipulation of the distended bowel should be kept to a minimum. If possible, the first step is to find collapsed bowel, and using bowel-grasping forceps, the bowel can be run proximally to the obstruction. Manipulation of the distended bowel should be avoided if possible as it is very easy to make an enterotomy in the edematous and friable obstructed bowel.

Small Bowel Obstruction Secondary to Adhesions

Typically, the patient has had previous abdominal surgery and presents with crampy abdominal pain and vomiting. The diagnosis is made by three views of the abdomen (Xray) or CT scan of the abdomen. In most patients, the bowel obstruction will resolve spontaneously. In about 20–30% of the cases, surgery is necessary. If the small bowel obstruction does not resolve within 24–48 h, surgery should be considered. There may be some advantages with the laparoscopic approach with fewer wound-related problems and complications compared to the open approach [3]. Table 10.1 illustrates a ten-step process for managing small bowel obstruction from adhesions.

There are two types of adhesive small bowel obstructions: single or a few bands and wide matted adhesions. Wide matted adhesions are typically more difficult to deal with but can still be managed laparoscopically. These kinds of dense adhesions are difficult to manage regardless of the approach (open or laparoscopic) and often take more time during dissection. If the surgeon realizes that the abdomen cavity is totally fused or frozen when placing the first port, pneumoperitoneum will unlikely be achieved resulting in unsafe visual exposure. Concern for patient safety should prompt the surgeon to proceed with laparotomy.

Table 10.1 Management of laparoscopic small bowel obstruction from adhesions

Step 1.	Select a safe entry point
Step 2.	Enter the abdomen safely
Step 3.	Lysis of adhesions to place ports
Step 4.	Sharp lysis of adhesions
Step 5.	Blunt lysis of adhesions
Step 6.	Avoid grasping dilated bowel
Step 7.	Identify non-dilated small bowel
Step 8.	Trace nondilated bowel to the site of obstruction
Step 9.	Divide the adhesion causing the obstruction
Step 10.	Inspect the small bowel at the site of obstruction and determine if resection is necessary

Small Bowel Obstruction from Hernias

Small bowel obstruction from an incarcerated hernia is a surgical emergency and should be done as soon as possible to reduce the risk of mortality [13]. Typically, a patient will present with a painful mass in the inguinal region, associated with nausea, vomiting, and crampy abdominal pain. The diagnosis is made on three views of the abdomen (Xray) or CT scan of the abdomen. The initial treatment should be nasogastric suction with intravenous fluids to replace estimated volume losses. Once the patient has been stabilized with adequate volume replacement, laparoscopic surgery can be performed [4].

The hernia can be reduced safely by pushing on the abdominal wall and gently trying to push the hernia contents back into the abdomen. Sometimes grasping the mesentery of the incarcerated bowel with gentle traction applied from inside the abdomen can facilitate reduction of the hernia. The distended and dilated small intestine should not be manipulated if possible, as this may easily lead to an enterotomy. If it is not possible to reduce the hernia contents in this manner, the surgeon can attempt to make the fascial opening larger by using cautery. Very often, by extending the opening of the hernia by 1 cm and then repeating the process of reducing the hernia by gentle pressure from the abdominal wall and gentle traction on the mesentery, this can result in a successful reduction of the hernia. The majority of incarcerated hernias can be reduced by using these maneuvers.

Once the hernia is reduced, the bowel must be carefully inspected. As in the open approach, the decision regarding the need for bowel resection should be based on the extent of ischemic injury and bowel viability. If a bowel resection and anastomosis is needed, this can be done extracorporeally through a minilaparotomy incision using a wound protector or intracorporeally depending on the surgeon's expertise and experience with laparoscopic bowel resections and anastomosis.

If no bowel resection is necessary, laparoscopic hernia repair can be performed. Other options for repairing the hernia would include primary repair without the use of mesh or a separate incision made through virgin territory with the use of a mesh. Another option would include repairing the hernia at a later date. The decision as to the hernia repair would depend on the stability of the patient, the degree of contamination, and the experience of the surgeon.

Food Bolus and Bezoar Obstruction

Often food bolus obstruction can present in a patient without previous surgery. If suspected, the patient can be treated with nasogastric suction and intravenous fluids. If the obstruction does not resolve within 24–48 h, surgery should be considered.

Often the diagnosis of food bolus obstruction can be made with CT scan. The principles of the surgery include identifying the site of obstruction laparoscopically and, if necessary, making a small laparotomy incision to milk the food bolus obstruction into the cecum. In patients who have a gastrectomy or gastric bypass, phytobezoars causing small bowel obstruction may be more common [12].

Gallstone Ileus

This diagnosis is usually made at the time of surgery. The patient may present with a small bowel obstruction with nausea, vomiting, and crampy abdominal pain. Gallstone ileus may be suspected on CT scan when gas is seen in the biliary tree [5]. At the time of surgery, the gallstone is removed through a small enterotomy and retrieved through one of the port sites. Alternatively, a small laparotomy can be performed to avoid peritoneal contamination. If there is evidence of ischemia, a bowel resection may be necessary. This can be done laparoscopically as well. The specimen may need to be removed through a small laparotomy incision, preferably with the use of a wound protector.

Foreign Bodies

Small bowel obstruction can be from foreign bodies such as a migrated stent [6]. The principles of nasogastric suction and intravenous fluids apply. Once the patient is resuscitated, surgery can be performed. In the case of a large foreign body such as a stent, a small Pfannenstiel or midline incision may be is necessary to safely remove the stent.

Tumors Causing Small Bowel Obstruction

The most common cause of a small bowel obstruction from a tumor is usually a carcinoma of the cecum presenting as a small bowel obstruction. The diagnosis is confirmed on CT scan of the abdomen showing a tumor in the cecum with a small bowel obstruction. The patient may present with crampy abdominal pain, nausea, and vomiting. In advanced malignancy causing small bowel obstruction, sometimes laparoscopic enterocolostomy can be used for palliation [7]. The treatment involves nasogastric suction, intravenous fluids, and resuscitation of the patient. Once the patient has stabilized, surgery should be performed. The treatment could involve laparoscopic ileostomy, laparoscopic right colon resection with primary ileocolic anastomosis, or ileocolostomy to bypass the obstruction.

Postoperative Bowel Obstruction

If bowel obstruction occurs within a few days of laparoscopic surgery, the initial treatment involves nasogastric suction and intravenous fluids. It is sometimes difficult to determine whether there is an ileus or a mechanical small bowel obstruction. Postoperative small bowel obstructions often warrant a CT scan to help determine the etiology such as a mechanical bowel obstruction (from an inadvertent stitch or port-site incarceration), ileus, hematoma, or abscess. An ileus may be managed conservatively with nasogastric suction and intravenous fluids and should resolve within a few days. Because laparoscopic surgery is associated with less inflammatory reaction when compared to open surgery, it is generally safer and easier to perform a laparoscopy exploration in the immediate postoperative period [10]. Postoperative bowel obstruction can be more serious after certain operations such as gastric bypass and should prompt an urgent laparoscopic intervention.

Small Bowel Obstruction Following Gastric Bypass

When a patient presents with a small bowel obstruction months or years after gastric bypass, the small bowel obstruction should be treated surgically. Commonly the cause is from an internal hernia [11]. If left, the consequences can be devastating as it may lead to bowel infarction and death. Very often, the patient will present with crampy abdominal pain, with a CT scan and an abdominal Xray that are reported as normal. Any patient who presents with crampy abdominal pain after gastric bypass should be considered for diagnostic laparoscopy to exclude small bowel obstruction.

Complications

Although there is increasing evidence to suggest that laparoscopic lysis of adhesions for small bowel obstruction will decrease complications, shorten hospital stay, and decrease healthcare costs compared with open lysis of adhesions [15], randomized controlled studies are lacking. According to the American College of Surgeons National Surgical Quality Improvement Project (NSQIP) database [14], the portion of small bowel obstruction treated laparoscopically has increased from 17.2% in 2006 to 28.7% in 2013. Open lysis of adhesions typically takes longer (66 versus 60 min, $P < 0.001$) with a longer hospital stay (8.9 versus 4.2 days, $P < 0.001$). Open lysis of adhesions has higher postsurgical complication rates when compared to laparoscopic lysis of adhesions [14, 15].

Take-Home Messages

1. Depending on patient factors (how critically ill the patient is) and the technical skills of the surgeon, a laparoscopic approach to the management of small bowel obstructions can be safely done.

2. Appropriate patient selection is key to ensure successful outcome of a minimally invasive approach to small bowel obstruction.

3. Nasogastric decompression and adequate resuscitation are essential before commencing a laparoscopic exploration for bowel obstruction.

4. Special attention to patient positioning, initial port access (open vs Veress), use of atraumatic graspers for mesentery and collapsed bowel, and cautery will help prevent unwanted serious complications.

References

1. O'Connor DB, Winter DC. The role of laparoscopy in the management of acute small-bowel obstruction: a review of over 2,000 cases. Surg Endosc. 2012;26(1):12–7. doi:10.1007/s00464-011-1885-9. Epub 2011 Sep 5.

2. Ghosheh B, Salameh JR. Laparoscopic approach to acute small bowel obstruction: review of 1061 cases. Surg Endosc. 2007;21(11):1945–1949. Epub 2007 Sep 19.

3. Sajid MS, Khawaja AH, Sains P, Singh KK, Baig MK. A systematic review comparing laparoscopic vs open adhesiolysis in patients with adhesional small bowel obstruction. Am J Surg. 2016;212(1):138–50. doi:10.1016/j.amjsurg.2016.01.030. Epub 2016 Apr 13.

4. Elnahas A, Kim SH, Okrainec A, Quereshy F, Jackson TD. Is laparoscopic repair of incarcerated abdominal hernias safe? Analysis of short-term outcomes. Surg Endosc. 2016;30(8):3262–6. doi:10.1007/s00464-015-4649-0. Epub 2015 Nov 5.

5. Zygomalas A, Karamanakos S, Kehagias I. Totally laparoscopic management of gallstone ileus – technical report and review of the literature. J Laparoendosc Adv Surg Tech A. 2012;22(3):265–8. doi:10.1089/lap.2011.0375. Epub 2012 Feb 3.

6. Quinn M, Luke D. Oesophageal stent migration following Billroth I gastrectomy: an unusual cause of small bowel obstruction. J Surg Case Rep. 2013;2013(2):pii: rjt004. doi:10.1093/jscr/rjt004.

7. Ferguson HJ, Ferguson CI, Speakman J, Ismail T. Management of intestinal obstruction in advanced malignancy. Ann Med Surg (Lond). 2015;4(3):264–70. doi:10.1016/j.amsu.2015.07.018. eCollection 2015.

8. Nordin A, Freedman J. Laparoscopic versus open surgical management of small bowel obstruction: an analysis of clinical outcomes. Surg Endosc. 2016. [Epub ahead of print].

9. Qureshi I, Awad ZT. Predictors of failure of the laparoscopic approach for the management of small bowel obstruction. Am Surg. 2010;76(9):947–50.

10. Goussous N, Kemp KM, Bannon MP, Kendrick ML, Srvantstyan B, Khasawneh MA, Zielinski MD. Early postoperative small bowel obstruction: open vs laparoscopic. Am J Surg. 2015;209(2):385–90. doi:10.1016/j.amjsurg.2014.07.012. Epub 2014 Oct 13.

11. Geubbels N, Röell EA, Acherman YI, Bruin SC, van de Laar AW, de Brauw LM. Internal herniation after laparoscopic Roux-en-Y gastric bypass surgery: pitfalls in diagnosing and the introduction of the AMSTERDAM classification. Obes Surg. 2016;26(8):1859–66. doi:10.1007/s11695-015-2028-5.

12. Parsi S, Rivera C, Vargas J, Silberstein MW. Laparoscopic-assisted extirpation of a phytobezoar causing small bowel obstruction after Roux-en-Y laparoscopic gastric bypass. Am Surg. 2013;79(2):E93–5.

13. Nilsson H, Nilsson E, Angerås U, Nordin P. Mortality after groin hernia surgery: delay of treatment and cause of death. Hernia. 2011;15(3):301–7. doi:10.1007/s10029-011-0782-4. Epub 2011 Jan 26.

14. Pei KY, Asuzu D, Davis KA. Will laparoscopic lysis of adhesions become the standard of care? Evaluating trends and outcomes in laparoscopic management of small-bowel obstruction using the American College of Surgeons National Surgical Quality Improvement Project Database. Surg Endosc. 2016. [Epub ahead of print].

15. Byrne J, Saleh F, Ambrosini L, Quereshy F, Jackson TD, Okrainec A. Laparoscopic versus open surgical management of adhesive small bowel obstruction: a comparison of outcomes. Surg Endosc. 2015;29(9):2525–32. doi:10.1007/s00464-014-4015-7. Epub 2014 Dec 6.

Benjamin Braslow

Introduction

The vermiform appendix, once thought to be a vestigial organ in humans, is a true diverticulum of the cecum (containing all layers of the colonic wall from mucosa to serosa) whose orifice is located at the base of the cecum, just caudad to the ileocecal valve where the three tenia coli converge. The average length of the appendix in adults is 9 cm, and the upper limit of normal for the transverse diameter is considered 6–7 mm. Although the base of the appendix is an anatomic constant, the tip can migrate to a retrocecal (64%), subcecal (32%), preileal (1%), postileal (0.5%), or pelvic position (2%). The appendiceal artery, a terminal branch of the ileocolic artery, courses through the mesoappendix and usually terminates at the appendiceal tip. We now know that the lymphoid pulp containing B and T lymphoid cells in the appendiceal lamina propria plays an active role in secretion of immunoglobulins, especially IgA and that the appendix likely also serves as a depot for normal colonic flora that may play a particular role in preventing *C. difficile* colitis following antibiotic exposure.

Appendicitis is considered the most common acute abdominal emergency requiring surgery. Roughly 300,000 patients per year are diagnosed with acute appendicitis in the USA, and it consumes ~1million hospital days per year. Appendicitis occurs most frequently in the second and third decades of life. In the USA, men have a lifetime incidence of ~8.5% vs. ~6.5% for women, and the most common cause is luminal obstruction with a fecalith or appendicolith. In younger patients, lymphoid hyperplasia is thought to be a more common etiology. Parasitic infections and neoplasm are less common causes. Regardless of the cause, the patho-

physiology of acute appendicitis is fairly constant. Luminal obstruction leads to progressive mucosal inflammation and secretion that has no outflow. This in turn leads to increased intraluminal pressure and distention which stimulates autonomic visceral pain afferent fibers clinically resulting in periumbilical discomfort unrelated to activity or position and usual anorexia. Once intraluminal pressure exceeds venous pressures, mucosal engorgement develops followed by progressive arterial inflow decline, and mucosal integrity is compromised. Transmural inflammation and bacterial invasion (most commonly *E.* coli and *Bacteroides* species) then develop, and depending on the anatomic location of the appendix and the peritoneal surface that comes in contact with the inflamed appendix, localized somatic pain fibers are stimulated and the pain migrates to that area, most commonly the right lower quadrant at McBurney's point. If this process is not mitigated either by spontaneous resolution of obstruction, antibiotics to slow the progression of bacterial-induced inflammation, or surgical removal, full thickness necrosis may develop, and the appendix is at risk for perforation. This can lead to contained abscess, local phlegmon, or at worst free spillage and diffuse peritonitis!

Preoperative Diagnostic Options

Subjective complaints and physical exam findings can be quite variable depending upon the anatomic location of the inflamed appendix and the degree of inflammation. An inflamed appendix adjacent to the anterior parietal peritoneum will present with classic right lower quadrant pain, maximal at McBurney's point often associated with focal rebound and guarding. In this patient, however, a positive "obturator sign" (pain elicited in the supine patient with passive internal rotation of the flexed right thigh) or a positive "psoas sign" (pain with passive extension of the right thigh in a patient placed in a left lateral recumbent position) might be absent.

B. Braslow (✉)
PENN Presbyterian Medical Center, Division of Trauma, Surgical Critical and Emergency Surgery, Philadelphia, PA, USA
e-mail: Benjamin.Braslow@uphs.upenn.edu

© Springer International Publishing AG 2018
K.A. Khwaja, J.J. Diaz (eds.), *Minimally Invasive Acute Care Surgery*, https://doi.org/10.1007/978-3-319-64723-4_11

Common laboratory findings in patients with acute appendicitis include a mild leukocytosis with or without a clear left shift and an elevated C-reactive protein (CRP) level. The diagnostic accuracy of these two studies is only moderate when considered individually, but sensitivity improves significantly in combination.

Currently, the modified Alvarado score is considered the most widely used clinical scoring system to identify patients with a high likelihood of an acute appendicitis as their source of abdominal pain. This system assigns a score to each of the following diagnostic criteria:

- Migratory right lower quadrant pain (1 point)
- Anorexia (1 point)
- Nausea or vomiting (1 point)
- Tenderness in the right lower quadrant to palpation (2 points)
- Rebound tenderness in the right lower quadrant (1 point)
- Fever >37.5 °C (>99.5 °F) (1 point)
- Leukocytosis of WBC >10 × 10⁹/L (2 points)

A patient's overall score is derived by summing the individual points. A score of <4 has been found to be a fairly good negative indicator for the diagnosis of acute appendicitis as the source of abdominal pain. The reality of today is that regardless of clinical suspicion, most individuals seen in a hospital emergency department for abdominal pain will undergo some form of diagnostic imaging to either confirm a suspected diagnosis or look for the clear source. This usually occurs prior to surgical consultation. The days of accepting a 15% negative appendectomy rate at the time of surgery are far gone. Modern imaging availability and accuracy appear to have reduced that rate to far less than 10%, and likely this number will continue to fall.

At present, computed tomography (CT) is recommended as the preferred imaging modality in the evaluation of suspected appendicitis in adults (overall sensitivity of 0.94 and specificity of 0.95). Ultrasound and MRI, which demonstrate lower diagnostic accuracy and higher operator variability than CT, are usually reserved for radiosensitive populations such as pregnant women and children. Intravenous contrast is recommended in CT exams performed for the diagnosis of appendicitis as it also improves the delineation of phlegmon or abscess if present. In patients with renal insufficiency or a history of moderate to severe hypersensitivity reaction to iodinated contrast, non-contrasted CT is an acceptable alternative with more than adequate sensitivity and specificity. The use of oral contrast can improve the accuracy of CT to rule out appendicitis, but this can delay the scan for several hours without a significant increase in sensitivity or specificity of the exam. Rectal contrast avoids the delay associated with oral administration but is usually not well tolerated or appreciated by the patient. Pertinent findings on CT include:

- An enlarged appendiceal diameter >6 mm with an occluded lumen
- Appendiceal wall thickening (>2 mm)
- Periappendiceal fat stranding
- Appendiceal wall enhancement (with IV contrast administration)
- Appendicolith (25% of patients)

Management of Presumed Uncomplicated Appendicitis

Traditionally, urgent appendectomy (usually within a 6–12 h window from presentation) has been the standard of care for the treatment of acute uncomplicated appendicitis. Recently, a paradigm shift to nonoperative management with antibiotic therapy alone has gained some popularity, and there are a plethora of studies looking at short- and long-term outcomes including failure rates and recurrence rates. For now, however, the American College of Surgeons, the Society for Surgery of the Alimentary Tract, and the World Society of Emergency Surgery still recommend appendectomy as the treatment of choice for acute uncomplicated appendicitis (without abscess or phlegmon). The most common reasons cited include:

1. Appendectomy can generally be performed with low morbidity and very low mortality.
2. Long-term recurrence rates following nonoperative management approach 15–25% and even higher in patients with fecaliths identified on imaging.
3. The risk of unexpected lesions in the appendix like carcinoid tumors or other malignancies is not zero and in fact increases to important levels with increases in age.
4. The cost of prolonged hospitalization for observation of the patient being managed with antibiotics, serial abdominal exams, and serial laboratory assessment can easily exceed the cost of early operative management followed by early (often same day) discharge.

Once the decision to operate has been made, the surgical technique used (open vs. laparoscopic) should be based on the surgeon's level of experience and comfort with either procedure and the institutional capabilities. The largest meta-analysis of recent data comparing the open vs. laparoscopic approach published by the Cochrane Collaboration showed that compared to the open technique, the laparoscopic appendectomy:

1. Reduced the risk of abdominal wall wound infection
2. Slightly increased the risk of intra-abdominal abscess
3. Took ~10 min longer
4. Caused less pain POD #1

5. Decreased hospital length of stay (LOS) by ~1.1 day
6. Had higher costs of operation but reduced overall hospital costs

Laparoscopic appendectomy has been shown to be the clear procedure of choice for certain patient populations. Included here are patients with an uncertain diagnosis as it allows for the inspection of other abdominal organs. This benefit may be greatest for women of childbearing age with a host of other potential pelvic pathologies that could cause right lower quadrant pain. Obese patients, where larger, morbidity-prone incisions might be needed to gain access to the appendix, also benefit from the laparoscopic approach. The last group for which the laparoscopic approach has shown a clear advantage is the elderly who had their hospital length of stay significantly lowered and discharge rates to home vs. some other facility significantly raised by the minimally invasive technique.

Operative Technique for Laparoscopic Appendectomy

In preparation for performing a laparoscopic appendectomy, the anesthetized patient is positioned supine on the operative table with his/her left arm, or both arms if body habitus allows, tucked (Fig. 11.1). The bladder should be decompressed either with a Foley catheter or by having the patient spontaneously void immediately prior to entering the operating room. This will serve to prevent bladder injury during suprapubic port placement. The abdomen is prepped from xiphoid to the pubis. We recommend that the initial port placed into the abdomen is a 12 mm blunt Hassan trocar placed via direct cutdown through a supraumbilical fold curvilinear incision. S-retractors are used to dissect down through the subcutaneous fat until the fascia at the linea alba is exposed. Kocher clamps are then used to grab the fascia bilaterally and tent it upward. A small vertical incision is

Fig. 11.1 Patient positioning. (1) Left arm tucked, right arm can be extended. (2) Foley catheter. (3) Surgeon and assistant on patient's left. (4) Video monitor on patient's right. (5) Intended port sites labeled

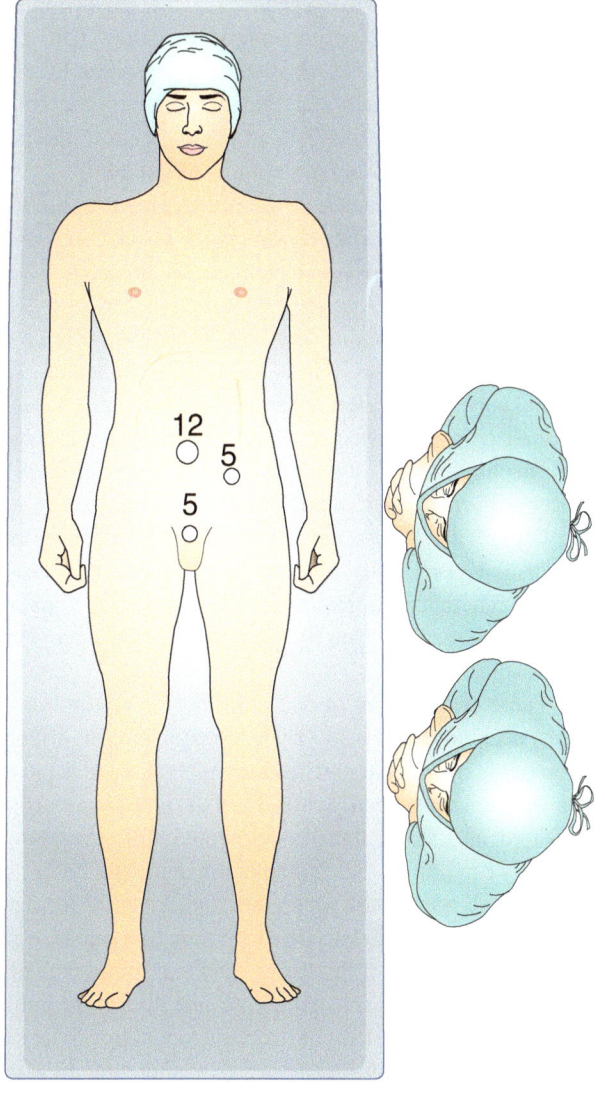

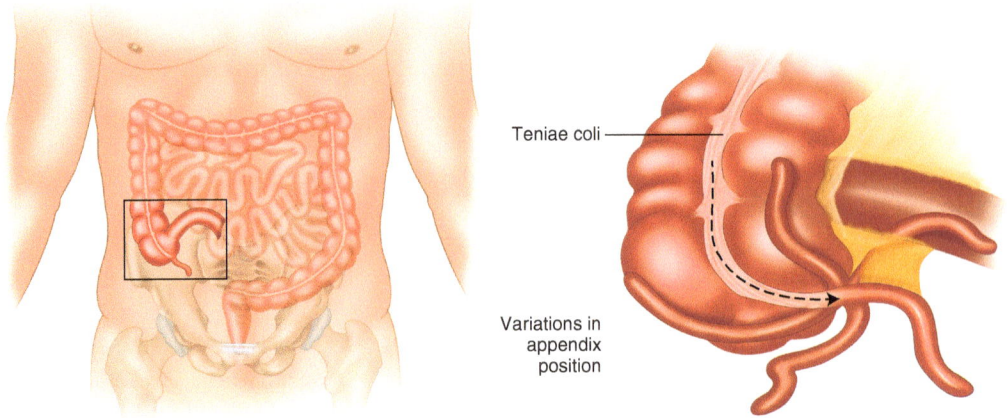

Teniae coli

Variations in
appendix
position

Fig. 11.2 Variations of appendiceal position. Best method of finding non-obvious appendix is to identify antimesenteric tenia and follow distally to appendiceal base where three tenias coalesce

then made in the fascia with a #15 blade, and the S-retractors are utilized again to dissect through the preperitoneal fat until the glistening peritoneum is exposed. Thin tipped hemostats are then used to grasp the peritoneum bilaterally and tent this layer upward; Metzenbaum scissors are then used to incise the peritoneum and gain access to the peritoneal cavity. At this time, stay sutures (usually 0-0 Vicryl) are then placed into the apices of the fascia. These are left untied and will be used during fascial closure at the conclusion of the operation. The Kocher clamps and the hemostats are removed, and the fascial opening is then probed with a finger to dilate up the opening and feel for any local adhesions. Next the blunt Hassan port is passed into the abdomen, the fascial stay sutures are wrapped around its ridged adjustable suture anchoring device, and pneumoperitoneum is achieved by attaching the CO_2 tubing and insufflating with high flow to a pressure of 12–15 mmHg.

Use of the Veress needle for initial port placement is acceptable (especially in a virgin abdomen), but there are certain inherent risks involved based on the blinded nature of this technique that can be avoided with the open Hassan approach.

There are a variety of port placement configurations that have been advocated, all of which emphasize the triangulation of the instrument ports and the appendix. Once pneumoperitoneum has been achieved, a 5 mm laparoscope is inserted into the abdomen, and exploratory laparoscopy is initially performed, taking note of inflammatory findings and abdominal adhesions which may alter trocar placement plans. Next under direct vision, a 5 mm port is placed in the left lower quadrant followed by a second 5 mm port placed under direct vision in the midline just above the pubis. A laparoscopic instrument may be used to tent up on the suprapubic midline peritoneum at the site of supraumbilical trocar placement to minimize injury to the underlying small bowel or colon in very close approximation to the usually compressible abdominal wall at this site. Both the operating surgeon and the assistant are now both situated on the patient's left. The laparoscope is then moved to the left lower quadrant trocar, and laparoscopic graspers are placed in the other ports as the patient is placed in steep Trendelenburg position, and the operating table is also partially rotated to the patient's left side. These bed maneuvers serve to help clear small bowel loops and omentum from the right lower quadrant to make identifying the appendix easier.

Using atraumatic graspers, the cecum is grasped, elevated, and sequentially followed to the point where the three tenias converge at its base which should correspond with the base of the appendix (Figs. 11.2 and 11.3). Once the diseased appendix is identified, any and all adhesions to surrounding structures should be lysed with a combination of blunt and sharp dissection. In the case of a retrocecal appendix, the lateral peritoneal attachments, the white line of Toldt, must be divided to mobilize the cecum and expose the appendix. The appendix should be grasped ideally at its tip, unless too inflamed and at risk for perforation with manual manipulation, and elevated toward the anterior abdominal wall. Soft cotton tip (peanut) dissectors work well for atraumatic blunt dissection, and over the years, we have come to rely on using an ultrasonic scalpel device for hemostatic sharp dissection. This device affords you the ability to dissect tissue similar to a Maryland dissector as well as hemostatically cut tissue like a laparoscopic shear. Other laparoscopic vessel-sealing and dividing devices are available as well, but the working tips tend to be more blunt and less amenable to precise tissue dissection. Our practice has evolved from using an Endo GIA stapling device to transect the mesoappendix after a widow was created in the mesoappendix between the base of the

Fig. 11.3 Mobilizing appendix. Atraumatic grasper on the right (Endo Babcock or alligator jaw) grabbing antimesenteric tenia and elevating cecum anteriorly helping to identify appendix inferiorly

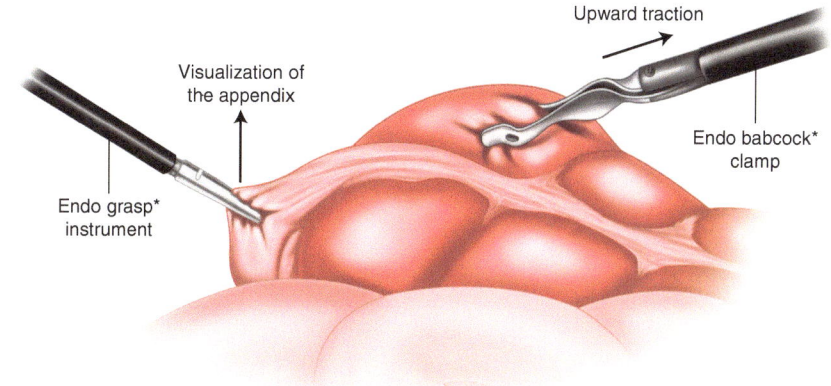

appendix and the cecum to simply using the ultrasonic scalpel device to transect the mesoappendix from its free edge to the appendiceal base (Fig. 11.4). Anecdotally we found that the Endo GIA stable lines were more prone to bleed postoperatively even if a white vascular load was utilized. There are alternative, cheaper means of transecting the mesoappendix (i.e., segmental laparoscopic clip placement and transection with endoshears), but this technique adds to the operative time as it requires more frequent instrument exchanges.

The appendiceal base is then transected off of the cecum using an Endo GIA stapling device with a blue staple load (Fig. 11.5). This device was brought into the abdomen through the umbilical 12 mm Hassan trocar. Ideally a small cuff of cecum is included with the specimen to ensure the entire appendix is included in the specimen and that the staples were placed in healthy, noninflamed tissue. This is especially important if the base of the appendix appears significantly inflamed or possibly necrotic. Again, there are alternative, cheaper ways to divide the appendix off of the cecum (i.e., division between endo-loops), but again this technique adds to operative time and leaves a cut edge of mucosa which requires fulguration and can increase abscess rates.

Rarely, if the tip and/or body of the appendix is too mired down in inflammatory adhesions, the base can be transected off of the cecum first, and the mesoappendix can be divided in any direction (free edge to base or vice versa). Occasionally, a third 5 mm trocar needs to be added for retraction purposes or simply to allow for a better angle of attack on the mesoappendix. This port is often needed in the right upper quadrant and can be placed and utilized with minimal or no added postoperative pain or morbidity.

If free or loculated purulent fluid is encountered intra-abdominally during appendiceal mobilization, it is best handled with primary suction clearance via a suction/irrigation

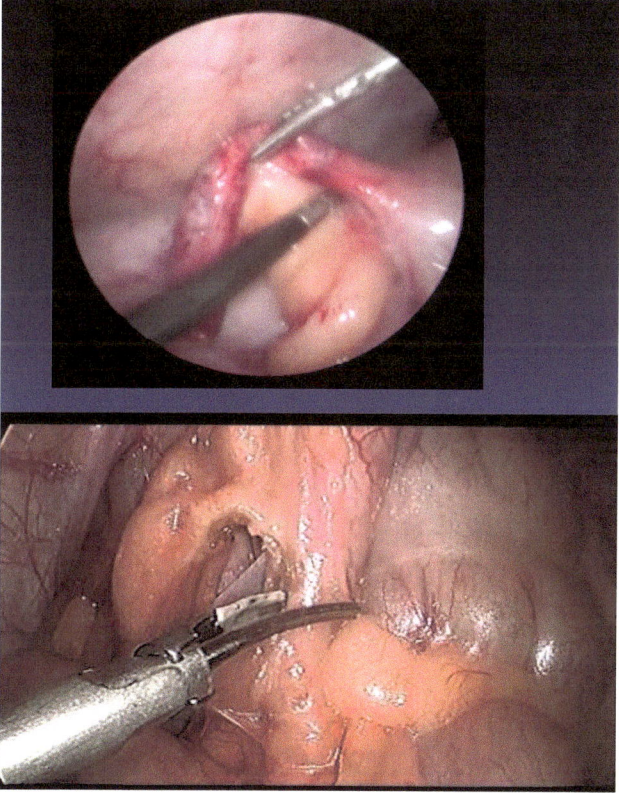

Fig. 11.4 Dividing mesoappendix with ultrasonic scalpel device. Taking mesoappendix from free edge to base of appendix with small sequential bites with ultrasonic scalpel

device and adequate but not excessive irrigation. Interestingly, in uncomplicated appendicitis, irrigation has been counterintuitively associated with higher intra-abdominal abscess rates in the laparoscopic approach. This is likely secondary to dissemination of contaminated fluid outside the right lower quadrant especially while the patient is in steep Trendelenburg position. Also, placement of postoperative

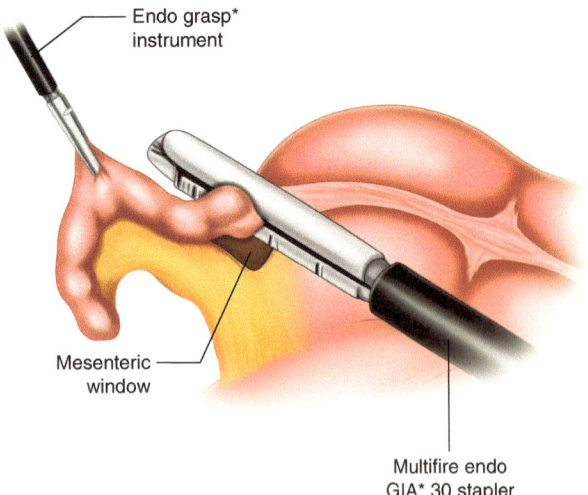

Fig. 11.5 Transection of appendix off of the cecum. Endo GIA stapler transecting appendix with small cuff of cecal tissue attached to base of the appendix

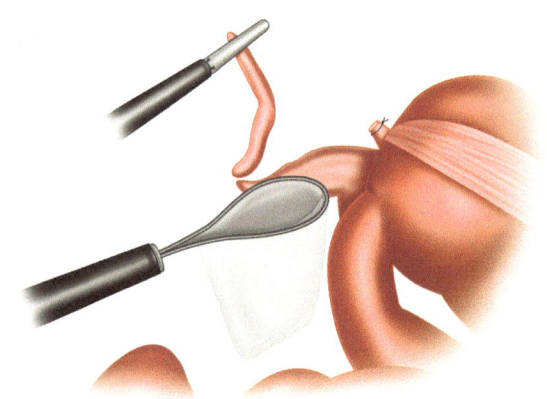

Fig. 11.6 Use of Endo Catch bag for removal of appendix to lower the chance of postoperative umbilical port site infection

peritoneal drains in appendectomies for uncomplicated appendicitis has never been shown to reduce the incidence of postoperative abscess, and in theory the negative pressure tubing near mesoappendiceal or cecal staple lines can be associated with higher rates of bleeding or staple line leaks.

Once completely freed of all adhesions and attachments, the appendix is placed in a laparoscopic specimen bag delivered intra-abdominally via the Hassan port and left in the abdominal cavity for eventual removal at the time of trocar removal (Fig. 11.6). Use of this bag helps minimize the risk of postoperative wound infection by direct contamination from the infected specimen.

If a normal-appearing appendix is identified during laparoscopy, a quick exploration of other pelvic structures should be carried out looking for another source of pain or inflammation (i.e., a fallopian tube or ovarian process, uter-

ine pathology, sigmoid colon diverticulitis, stigmata of Crohn's disease on terminal ilium, cecum, etc.). If an obvious source other than the appendix (and not involving the appendix) is identified, a normal appendix can be left in situ and the other process addressed. If no other source is obvious, the normal-appearing appendix should be removed. This will take the appendix out of the differential diagnosis as the cause of subsequent presentations with right lower quadrant pain, and often the pathology of the normal-appearing appendix will indeed show some inflammatory changes. In the setting of unexpected findings of terminal ileitis with or without other stigmata of Crohn's disease, special consideration must be given to performing the intended appendectomy because of a higher likelihood of postoperative fistula formation. In general, if the appendix appears uninvolved in the inflammatory process, it may be safely removed, again, to help avoid future diagnostic conundrums. If extensive involvement of the cecum or appendiceal base is identified, the appendix should be left in situ with the rest of the inflammatory process for subsequent medical treatment of presumed Crohn's disease.

An indication for conversion to an open procedure would be in this setting of suspected Crohn's disease, where a perforation of the ileum, cecum, or appendix is appreciated and ileocecectomy is deemed necessary for source control.

Postoperative Concerns

The most common complication following laparoscopic appendectomy is infection, either a wound infection (usually at the umbilical port site) or an intra-abdominal abscess. Usually these complications are limited to patients who were found to have evidence of perforation intraoperatively. Wound infections can usually be managed with antibiotic treatment +/− wound opening and drainage. Intra-abdominal abscess usually requires placement of a percutaneous drain under CT or ultrasound guidance. Unfortunately, both of these complications are often discovered after the patient has been discharged home and prompt return visits to the emergency department for evaluation and probable admission. If perforation and significant contamination were discovered at the time of surgery, the operative surgeon might consider a short course (24–48 h) of postoperative IV antibiotics (not indicated in cases of uncomplicated appendicitis) and a lengthier period of observation prior to the usual discharge within 24 h from surgery. In these patients, postoperative ileus is also more common and may require a delay in starting regular diet.

Any patient with hemodynamic instability in the early postoperative period should be evaluated for the possibility of an intra-abdominal bleeding source. Serial hemoglobin/hematocrit levels should be sent and serial abdominal exams performed looking for distention and increased pain. Laboratory, radiographic, or physical evidence of bleeding should prompt immediate return to OR for laparoscopic exploration and identification and control of bleeding source usually present within the remnant mesoappendix.

The pathology of the removed appendix must be checked as the incidence of neoplastic disease can be as high as 1%. Carcinoid tumors account for nearly two thirds of all appendiceal neoplasms, but others including mucinous cystadenoma, mucinous cystadenocarcinoma, non-mucinous adenocarcinoma (i.e., signet ring cell), or appendiceal lymphoma could be identified, and consultation with a surgical oncologist should be suggested.

Management of Perforated Appendicitis

For the patient diagnosed with a perforated appendicitis by preoperative imaging, immediate surgical intervention can be associated with greater than a threefold increase in postoperative morbidity compared to nonoperative management. For this reason, the treatment algorithm for known perforated complicated appendicitis contains two arms: one for patients with septic physiology and generalized peritonitis and the other for patients with hemodynamic stability and evidence of a localized inflammatory process (i.e., contained abscess or phlegmon). The former require aggressive volume resuscitation, broad-spectrum antibiotic administration, and prompt surgical exploration for control of contamination. This surgery may take the form of an open exploratory laparotomy with ileocecal resection +/− ileocecal anastomosis or end ileostomy/colonic mucous fistula creation depending on the degree of contamination and the patient's hemodynamic status. Newer practices take a much less invasive approach to this patient population by scaling down the initial operation to either laparoscopic or open drainage, adequate washout, and strategic drain placement alone without formal resection to achieve source control and allow for mitigation of the driving inflammatory source with subsequent antibiotic therapy.

The latter group with contained abscess and phlegmon in the current management paradigm is treated with either IV antibiotic therapy alone as for pure phlegmon vs. IV antibiotics or percutaneous drainage if abscess is present.

The practice of interval laparoscopic appendectomy is currently a topic of hot debate in the literature. For adult patients who are successfully treated nonoperatively, there is a low risk of developing a recurrent appendicitis. This risk substantially increases in the presence of a fecalith identified on initial imaging. Also the risk of missing an underlying condition such as inflammatory bowel disease or a neoplasm

Take-Home Messages
1. Subjective complaints and physical exam findings can be quite variable depending upon the anatomic location of the inflamed appendix and the degree of inflammation.
2. CT scan is recommended as the preferred imaging modality in the evaluation of suspected appendicitis in adults (overall sensitivity of 0.94 and specificity of 0.95), and wide-scale usage has greatly decreased the incidence of negative appendectomy.
3. Port placement during laparoscopic appendectomy can vary but should always emphasize the triangulation of the instrument ports and the appendix.
4. The ultrasonic scalpel device works exceptionally well as both a dissecting instrument (freeing up periappendiceal adhesions) and a tissue sealant during transection of the mesoappendix.
5. In laparoscopic appendectomies for uncomplicated appendicitis, irrigation and drain placement are not only unnecessary but may also be associated with higher rates of postoperative abscess and or bleeding.
6. In contrast to above, damage control laparoscopic techniques including abdominal washout and suction drain placement can be utilized in the operative treatment of a hemodynamically unstable patient with diffuse peritonitis from an unresectable inflamed/perforated appendix.

increases with age. It seems appropriate to recommend laparoscopic interval appendectomy for adult patients over 40 years of age and to obtain a screening colonoscopy prior to surgery. Surgery should be delayed for a minimum of 8 weeks following resolution of symptoms after drainage and/or antibiotic therapy.

Key References

1. Sauerland S, Jaschinski T, Neugebaur EA. Laparoscopic versus open surgery for suspected appendicitis. Cochrane Database Syst Rev. 2010;10:CD001546.
2. Korndorffer JR Jr, Fellinger E, Reed W. SAGES guideline for laparoscopic appendectomy. Surg Endosc. 2010;24(4):757–61. epub 2009.
3. Wright GP, Mater ME, Carroll JT, et al. Is there truly an oncologic indication for interval appendectomy? Am J Surg. 2015;209:442.
4. Garst GC, Moore EE, Banerjee MN, et al. Acute appendicitis: a disease severity score for the acute care surgeon. J Trauma Acute Care Surg. 2013;74:32.

Matthew Randall Rosengart

Introduction

Colonic diverticular disease, including diverticulosis and diverticulitis, continues to comprise a common clinical entity in the United States that imposes substantial economic burden and allocation of healthcare resources. The most recent analyses estimate that the diseases collectively account for a little over 300,000 annual hospital admissions that consume 1.5 million acute care bed days annually and cost upward of 2.5–3 billion dollars each year in the United States [1–3]. Contemporary analyses suggest that a more algorithmic acute care surgical approach, tailored to the specific phenotype of the interaction between patient and disease, may offer improved morbidity and mortality.

Pathophysiology and Epidemiology

Colonic diverticular disease is commonly characterized as left or right sided, as each is thought to represent a distinct pathophysiology and epidemiology. Westernized and developed societies possess high prevalences of left-sided disease, which comprises upward of 90% of cases [4, 5]. Studies highlight that with increasing industrialization, and its accompanying changes in longevity and diet (i.e., deficiency of dietary fiber), the prevalence of diverticular disease increases: 50–70% of individuals older than 80 years have diverticulosis, and 80% of cases of diverticulitis occur in individuals older than 50 years [2, 5, 6]. By contrast, right colonic disease typically occurs in subjects of Asian descent and is considered to be a consequence of genetic predisposition [2, 7]. Nonetheless, Asian populations still exhibit a higher prevalence of left-sided disease.

The pathology of colic diverticulosis is an outpouching of the mucosa and submucosa typically along the taenia. The entity is thought to be the collective consequence of three processes: (1) structural abnormalities of the colonic wall, (2) intestinal dysmotility, and (3) a deficiency of dietary fiber [2]. The structural strength of the colonic wall is weakest at segments parallel to the mesenteric taenia, where the vasa recta penetrate the circular muscle to supply the mucosa and submucosa [8]. Specimens from subjects with diverticulosis show an accordion-like effect called "concertina," due to a thickening of the circular muscle, a shortening of the taenia due to increased elastin content, and a narrowing of the luminal caliber [2, 9]. These anatomic alterations parallel perturbations in normal colonic physiology. The luminal pressures of subjects with sigmoid diverticulosis have been shown to be higher than basal levels of population controls [2, 10, 11]. Similar observations have been observed in cases of right-sided diverticular disease [2]. Studies utilizing cineradiography have observed disordered peristalsis in which haustral contractions occur simultaneously rather than sequentially [11]. The consequence is "segmentation" of the colon with regionally high pressures that are postulated to contribute to diverticulosis [11, 12]. This phenomenon has been correlated with diets in low fiber. Indeed this last association has received the greatest attention as a causal mechanism [2]. Collectively, the data are compelling that low dietary fiber contributes to the diverticulosis and, in fact, administration may be of benefit in managing the disease [13–16]. Fiber is thought to bulk stool volume, facilitate mass movement, and lower intracolonic pressures. Several studies have reported a negative association between dietary fiber intake and the development of diverticular disease, which has been recapitulated in mechanistic animal studies [14–16]. Additional factors proposed to contribute to diverticulosis include inflammation, smoking, obesity and a lack of physical activity, caffeine and alcohol consumption, and the use of nonsteroidal anti-inflammatory drugs [17–19].

M.R. Rosengart (✉)
Department of Surgery, University of Pittsburgh Medical Center, Pittsburgh, PA, USA
e-mail: rosengartmr@upmc.edu

© Springer International Publishing AG 2018
K.A. Khwaja, J.J. Diaz (eds.), *Minimally Invasive Acute Care Surgery*, https://doi.org/10.1007/978-3-319-64723-4_12

Clinical Presentation

Nearly one in four of patients with diverticular disease will present with symptoms of diverticulitis, and the risk of an episode correlates well with increasing age [2, 20]. Like most diseases the ultimate phenotype of the host-disease interaction occurs along a broad spectrum: from mild formes frustes to florid septic shock with multiple organ dysfunction. The modified classification scheme of Hinchey prognosticates morbidity and mortality and both the likelihood and choice of operative intervention (Table 12.1) [21, 22].

Acute, uncomplicated diverticulitis occurs in 75% of cases and refers to episodes of diverticular inflammation in the absence of intraperitoneal perforation, pericolonic abscess, hemorrhage, or stricture/obstruction. The classic triad of fever, leukocytosis, and right or left lower quadrant pain/tenderness occurs in the majority but does little to distinguish diverticulitis from other common pathologies: inflammatory bowel disease, acute appendicitis, urological and gynecological disorders, and colonic tumors. However, it should prompt tailored biochemical and hematologic analyses (i.e., complete blood count), a urinalysis, and radiographic evaluation with computed tomography (CT). The cumulative evidence highlights the near-perfect (~99%) sensitivity and (~99%) specificity of CT as a diagnostic tool for acute diverticulitis, the most frequent signs being colonic wall thickening and pericolonic fat stranding [23]. These data also underscore the merits of CT in identifying, qualifying, and quantifying complications, disease extent, and alternate pathology, such as adenocarcinoma.

Fifty to eighty percent of patients will respond to medical therapy, which typically involves either oral or parenteral antibiotics; some patients may require intravenous fluids. There are no data to support routine NPO status or NGT decompression for subjects with acute, uncomplicated diverticulitis, particularly in the absence of obstruction. A variety of antibiotic regimens are possible; however, the chosen regimen must ensure coverage of gram-negative and anaerobic coverage. A recent systematic review by the Surgical Infections Society (SIS) provides an exhaustive review and excellent guidance [24]. Despite appropriate antibiotics, in a significant minority of patients, symptoms will not completely resolve. Such circumstances should prompt follow-up CT imaging to evaluate for secondary complications. Abscess formation, extracolonic gas or contrast, and pneumoperitoneum are predictors of failure of medical management and indicate a high risk of secondary complications in the future.

Fifteen to twenty-five percent of patients will exhibit signs of complicated diverticulitis upon first presentation, which may necessitate procedural intervention on either an elective or urgent basis. Indications for urgent/emergent operation include free perforation with peritonitis, physiologic deterioration despite medical management, fistula formation, abscess not amenable to percutaneous drainage, and hemorrhage.

Perforation and Abscess Free perforation and peritonitis occur in < 20% of cases presenting to the hospital for management. The modified score of Hinchey (Table 12.1) provides accurate prognostication (i.e., morbidity, mortality) and an assessment of the need for operative intervention (Table 12.1). Patients with Hinchey III–IV should undergo operative intervention, and if permitting, laparoscopy should be the initial operative technique [25–27].

Abscess formation complicates approximately 10–20% of cases of diverticulitis: Hinchey Ia–II (Table 12.1). Initial diagnosis and management are similar to acute, uncomplicated diverticulitis. CT imaging provides invaluable information regarding abscess dimensions, location relative to other viscera, and thus the degree to which it is amenable to CT-guided percutaneous drainage. Medical management with or without percutaneous drainage is successful as the initial management for the majority (74–88%) of cases [21, 25]. However, it is currently perceived to indicate a more virulent process with a high risk of recurrence and complications. In one study, 60.5% of subjects initially successfully managed without surgery experienced recurrent diverticulitis, including 74% who had undergone percutaneous drainage [25]. Of recurrent cases, there was a high incidence of local disease complications, and nearly a third required an urgent operation. Similar conclusions were

Table 12.1 Modified Hinchey classification of diverticular disease [21

Stage	Modified Hinchey classification	CT findings	Mortality [5, 76]
Ia	Confined pericolic inflammation or phlegmon	Pericolic/peridiverticular fat stranding with adjacent colonic wall thickening	<5%
Ib	Pericolic or mesocolic abscess	Characteristics of Ia with abscess (<4 cm)	<5%
II	Pelvic, distant intra-abdominal, or retroperitoneal abscess	Characteristics of Ia and distant abscess (deep pelvic or peridiverticular/pericolic abscess >4 cm)	<5%
III	Generalized purulent peritonitis	Pneumoperitoneum with localized or generalized ascites with or without peritoneal wall thickening	13%
IV	Generalized fecal peritonitis	Amorphous, fecalized fluid/mass with open communication between bowel lumen and peritoneal cavity through the diverticulum	43%

reached in a systematic review of elective resection vs. observation after nonoperative management of complicated diverticulitis with abscess [26]. Thus, laparoscopic resection should be offered to subjects of appropriate risk/benefit ratios [27].

Fistula Colovesical and colovaginal fistulas comprise the majority of fistulas due to diverticular disease, the latter being more common in women who have undergone hysterectomy [28]. The clinical presentation of recurrent urinary tract infections or pneumaturia in the setting of diverticulosis is nearly diagnostic [29]. Cystoscopy is a commonly employed and highly accurate method of diagnosis, though a technique of poppy seed ingestion paired with subsequent urinalysis offers similar sensitivity [29]. After careful preoperative risk assessment and optimization, patients should be offered operative repair, which, though complex, can be accomplished via minimally invasive approaches [21, 27, 30, 31].

Gastrointestinal Hemorrhage Twenty to twenty-five percent of all cases of lower gastrointestinal bleeding are the consequence of colonic diverticula; and 17% of individuals with diverticulosis will experience hemorrhage [32, 33]. Hypertension, diabetes, coagulopathy, and ischemic heart disease are each considered predisposing causes. Patients typically present as painless melena (right-sided source) or maroon/red stool (left-sided source), though hemorrhage can be massive and culminate in hemorrhagic shock. In 60–90% of cases, bleeding spontaneously ceases, yet recurrence is reported in upward of 25% of cases [33, 34]. Caution should be exercised in interpreting these estimates as they potentially underestimate risk in the context of the increasing use of irreversible platelet and direct thrombin inhibitors. Efforts should be directed at the "ABCs" of resuscitation, localizing the source, ensuring hemostasis, and estimating the risk of recurrent hemorrhage and thus likelihood of operative intervention. Pharmacologic vitamin K antagonists (i.e., warfarin) can be rapidly reversed with either fresh frozen plasma or multifactor prothrombin complex concentrates (PCC) [35, 36]. PCC also exhibits some activity in reversing the newer direct thrombin inhibitors—rivaroxaban, apixaban, and edoxaban—a newer reversal agent for dabigatran that consists of a Fab fragment of a monoclonal antibody is available and effective: idarucizumab.

Numerous modalities exist for localizing the source, yet it is a fundamental component in patient care when view in the context that blind subtotal colectomy is associated with rebleeding rates as high as 20–40%. Colonoscopy has historically been the gold standard for localizing lower gastrointestinal hemorrhage, is safe, and offers therapeutic endoscopic therapy, even in studies restricted to diverticular hemorrhage [37–39]. Some studies suggest it may fail to identify the source in the absence of a bowel preparation, be

associated with increased risk of bleeding, and require additional intervention to control bleeding [40]. However, additional contemporary studies suggest that it reduces the allocations or resources, such as length of stay, and may provide quantification of risk of recurrent hemorrhage [40, 41]. The risk of rebleeding is not inconsequential (20–50%) and should prompt operative intervention [39, 42, 43]. A recent systematic review reported a high diagnostic accuracy of CT angiography for detecting and localizing active acute GI hemorrhage as low as 0.2 mL/min: sensitivity 85.2% (95% CI 75.5–91.5%) and specificity of 92.1% (95% CI 76.7–97.7%) [44]. Angiography also accurately localizes bleeding though is less sensitive at bleeding rates less than 1 mL/min. Furthermore, it is an invasive procedure with associated risks of contrast-induced kidney injury, allergic reaction, and vascular complications. However, angiography affords an opportunity for embolization, with reported initial success rates of 60–90% and applicability to management of the hemodynamically unstable patient [45–48]. Prior concerns about inducing mesenteric ischemia, infarction, and perforation have not borne out in observational trials [48, 49]. Recurrence occurs in approximately 20% and should prompt operative intervention [46–48].

Preoperative Preparation and Operative Intervention

Elective Resection

Elective surgery in the context of acute, uncomplicated diverticulitis (≤Hinchey Ia) is no longer routine practice even for young patients with minimal operative risk. In a multicenter retrospective analysis, the risk of recurrence was 13% after a median follow-up of nearly 9 years [50]. Similar conclusions were reported in a Markov probabilistic model: among younger subjects (<50 years) operative intervention after the fourth episode yielded a 0.1% fewer deaths and 2% fewer colostomies and saved over $5000 [51]. Similar results were obtained in a subcohort analysis of older subjects [51]. Despite these data, the surgical community is still slow to accept these recommendations as a follow-up nationwide analysis by the same group reported that nearly 95% of elective resections for acute uncomplicated diverticulitis occur after fewer than three episodes [52].

Though some debate persists regarding the necessity of elective resection in Hinchey I and II, the collective data do support higher recurrence and complication rates [25, 26]. Furthermore, increased risk of recurrence is associated for the previously described demographics and comorbidities (i.e., increasing age, obesity). Thus, elective operative intervention should be offered to those patients deemed to be of appropriate risk. The current literature strongly supports the superiority of laparoscopic resection and anastomosis over open laparotomy, as evidenced by reduced blood loss, reduced pain and perioperative analgesia, reduced complications (notably surgical site infections), and improved quality of life [53–55].

Operative Technique

All patients, elective or urgent, should undergo extensive preoperative risk assessment: optimization of comorbidities, ASA classification, and quantification of frailty [56–58]. Though a mechanical bowel preparation may facilitate bowel manipulation, the data do not otherwise support its sole use in reducing perioperative infectious complications [59]. Similarly there is equipoise regarding the use of oral antibiotics, though a recent meta-analysis suggests benefit in reducing SSI when combined with mechanical bowel preparation and systemic antibiotics [60]. All patients should receive preoperative and appropriately timed intraoperative antibiotics and a chlorhexidine-alcohol-based skin prep solution to optimally reduce the risk of surgical site infections [61, 62]. Sequential compression devices (SCDs) should be placed prior to induction of anesthesia, though it is the authors' preference to administer unfractionated subcutaneous heparin for venous thromboembolism prophylaxis. Patients should be positioned supine for right-sided disease and in modified lithotomy in approaching left-sided disease. Appropriately securing the patient to the operative table, including a footboard, will enable liberal use of extreme positioning (i.e., Trendelenburg), thereby allowing gravity to be utilized as an additional and useful retraction mechanism [63].

Port placement is tailored to the colonic segment to be resected and usually entails three to four trocars of 5-mm and 12-mm dimension (Fig. 12.1). As with all laparoscopic techniques, the principle tenets are triangulation and appropriate spacing of ports to (1) optimize direct access to target organs; (2) provide optimal vision of the operative field, thereby minimizing "sword fighting" and decreasing mental and muscular fatigue; and (3) enhance recognition of structures and minimize iatrogenic injury [64]. An excellent review by Ferzli and Fingerhut describes a simple standardized method of trocar placement for laparoscopic abdominal procedures: general estimation of port placement (Fig. 12.1a), right colon (Fig. 12.1b) and left/sigmoid colon (Fig. 12.1c) [64]. However, positioning an additional trocar lateral and in the midclavicular line may facilitate mobilization of the hepatic or splenic flexures (Figs. 12.1d, 12.1e).

The operative approach can be characterized as the following: medial to lateral, lateral to medial, superior to inferior, and inferior to superior [63]. The authors' preference is lateral to medial to enter the avascular retroperitoneal plane at the white line of Toldt [63, 65]. For both the right and left colon, dissection progresses medially to lift the entire colon segment up to the extent that it is truly at the abdominal median. A tension-free anastomosis necessitates release of the gastrocolic ligament and mobilization of the respective hepatic and splenic flexures. Care must be exercised to avoid dissecting deep into the retroperitoneal structures. With experience the pneumoperitoneum can be "harnessed" to facilitate dissection in the avascular retroperitoneal plane, thereby limiting the amount of "energy" needed for vascular control and protecting the ureters, vessels, and other structures (e.g., duodenum). Extensive repositioning of the table, and thereby the patient, will enable gravity to provide substantial retraction, e.g., steep Trendelenburg and right lateral decubitus clear the small bowel from the sigmoid and left colon. With this approach the specimen is mobilized toward the camera, which may progressively impede visualization and require moving the camera to an alternate port. The surgeon should become familiar operating in the setting of various camera angle perspectives (e.g., backward mirrored view). Similarly, the inflammation of diverticulitis can distort and ablate the typical anatomic planes and make dissection challenging; in such circumstances the surgeon should be prepared to utilize an alternate approach, including open exploration. Regardless of the initial approach, each can be continued upon conversion to an open technique, which is reported to occur in approximately 15% of cases due to inflammation, obfuscation of normal anatomy compromising safe dissection, iatrogenic injury, or inability to progress [65]. Recently, hand-assisted laparoscopic surgery (HALS) has been promoted as useful in complex dissections, to facilitate those less experienced in laparoscopy and avoid conversion to an open technique [66]. It has been shown to yield similar outcomes to procedures completed completely laparoscopic [66, 67].

Upon completion of visceral dissection, the proximal and distal margins are transected, which can be accomplished intra- or extracorporeally. It is imperative to ensure that all disease, to the extent safely possible, is removed and the remaining tissue margins are normal. Left-sided disease requires transecting the rectosigmoid junction at peritoneal reflection. Passing a 29 mm circular stapler to the level of the planned resection will enable the surgeon to assess whether or not the resection line is on the soft rectum [63]. The specimen is then extracted, and it is our practice to use a wound protector to minimize surgical site infection. For the right colon, a midline umbilical working incision is employed, as it typically is well positioned over the vascular pedicles of the afferent and efferent limbs and facilitates extracorporeal anastomosis (Fig. 12.1d) [63]. Alternatively, a transverse right upper quadrant or right lower quadrant site may be used [63]. For extraction of the left and sigmoid colon, a suprapubic working incision proves best, as it also enables an estimation of the sufficiency of mobilization of the proximal resection margin to ensure a tension-free anastomosis (Fig. 12.1e).

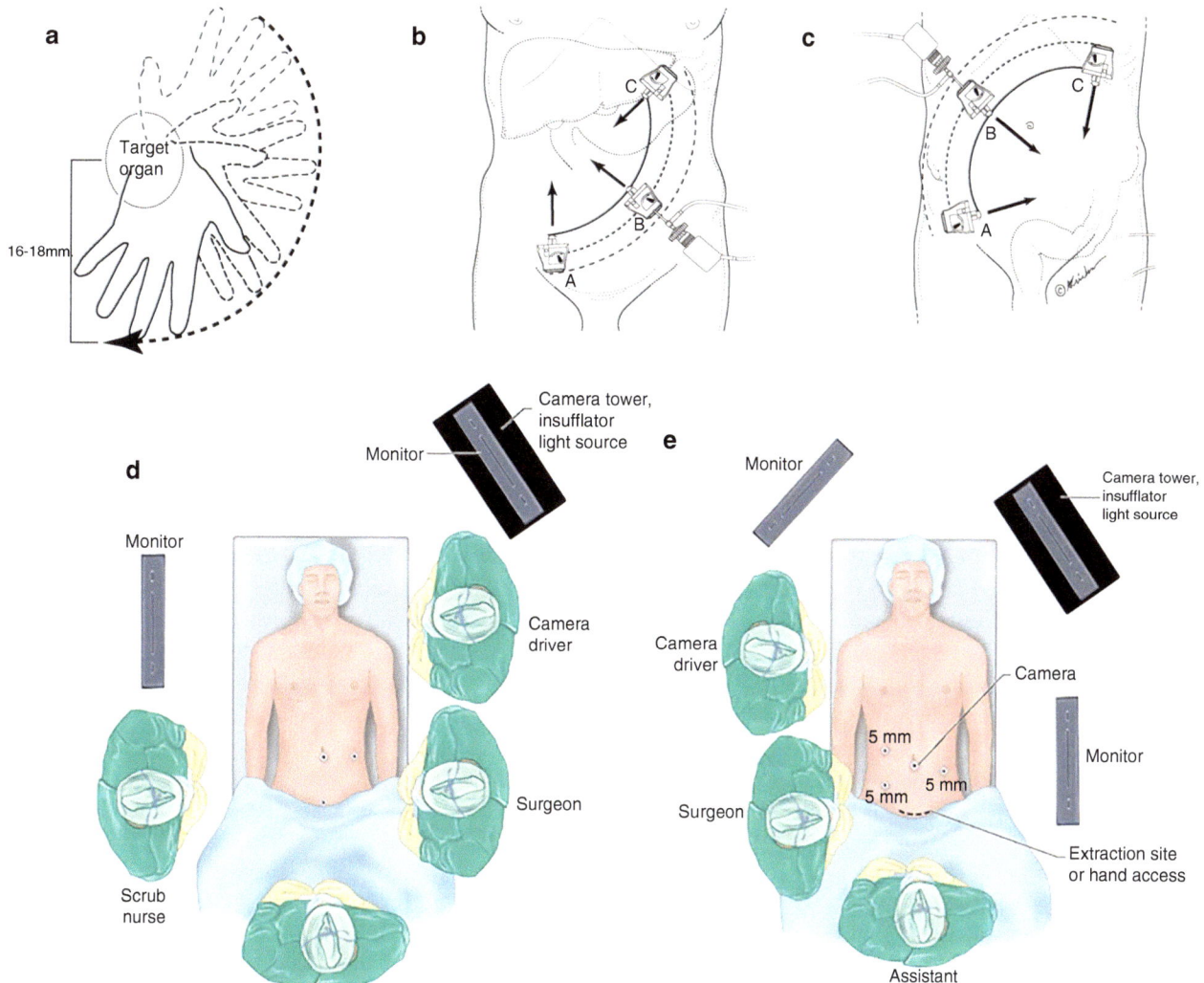

Fig. 12.1 (**a**) Method of estimating arc for trocar placement centered on target organ. (**b**) Trocar placement for right hemicolectomy. (**c**) Trocar placement for left/sigmoid hemicolectomy. (**d**) Alternate trocar placement and operative team positioning for right hemicolectomy. (**e**) Alternate trocar placement and operative team positioning for left hemicolectomy (This article was published in *Atlas of surgical techniques for colon, rectum, and anus*, Fleshman J, Jr., Birnbaum E, Hunt S, Mutch M, Kodner I, Safar B, Chapter 2, *Laparoscopic Right Colectomy*; Chapter 6, Laparoscopic Left Colectomy, Copyright Elsevier 2013)

In elective resections or in hemodynamically normal and stable urgent operations in non-frail patients without feculent peritonitis, where pliable soft proximal and distal bowel ends can be achieved, anastomosis may be performed. Stapled, hand-sewn, or a combination of methods may be utilized for construction of the anastomosis, and the principles of a tension-free anastomosis with preserved blood supply should be respected and maintained. There continues to be equipoise regarding the superiority of any one method, though recent data from studies of elective general surgery or of ileocolic anastomoses support stapled anastomoses in minimizing the risk of anastomotic leak [68–70]. In elective operations for diverticulitis, primary anastomosis is almost always achieved. The use of upstream fecal diversion with loop ileostomy may be used at the surgeon's discretion, such as in cases where extensive

inflammation or abscesses are encountered during the resection or anastomosis is less than ideal despite all efforts to achieve tension-free anastomosis of well-perfused ends. The adjunctive use of tools to assure adequate blood flow, such as the use of intravenous isocyanine green and fluorescent evaluation, may be useful to minimize the chance of anastomotic failure.

Several key principles should be practiced to the point of habit. Utilize only blunt and atraumatic instruments, including a Babcock grasper. Even with this precaution, minimize direct grasping of the bowel; rather gently lift, sweep, push, or suspend it. During sharp dissection, be continually cognizant of the structures residing behind any incision being made. All devices used for dissection and vessel control are sufficient (i.e., radiofrequency, harmonic, mechanical stapler), yet the operator should be familiar with the specific advantages and limitations of each. When dividing a vessel, ensure that an alternate means of control is readily available if the initial sealing device fails. A smoke evacuator or an insufflator system, which functions at a high enough volume, is essential to remove the plume generated by energy devices.

Emergent surgery in acute complicated diverticulitis (Hinchey III and IV) may also proceed with either laparoscopy or an open approach, depending upon patient physiology and preoperative assessment of operative complexity (e.g., prior laparotomy). Bear in mind that in the context of severe sepsis or septic shock, expeditious and definitive source control is the priority, which in some settings of operative difficulty or based upon surgeon experience may be best achieved by open approach.

Preoperatively a patent airway and ventilation are ensured, and appropriate central venous and arterial lines are placed for hemodynamic monitoring and resuscitation. Laparoscopy proceeds as previously described, though the ultimate goals are tailored, dictated in large part by patient physiology. In either open or laparoscopic approaches, resection of the perforation-bearing segment of the colon is the preferred procedure, rather than the entire disease-bearing segment once the decision has been made to forgo anastomosis and to perform a colostomy and close of the distal rectum (Hartmann's procedure). Mobilization of the colonic flexures is postponed if possible, so as to preserve the native tissue planes and facilitate dissection at the subsequent operation to restore intestinal continuity.

In cases of urgent operative management of Hinchey III or less, the reported trend is to advocate for definitive resection with colorectal anastomosis, with or without loop ileostomy. Though the data support ileocolonic anastomosis as the standard of care for right-sided complicated diverticulitis, whether to proceed with primary anastomosis or Hartmann's procedure at the index operation for left-sided disease is an area of ongoing debate. In the absence of persistent distributive shock, coagulopathy, and organ dysfunction, the evidence does support that primary anastomosis with or without proximal diverting ileostomy is safe and may reduce morbidity and mortality and improve quality of life [71, 72]. This should not be considered in hemodynamically unstable patients, frail patients that would poorly tolerate the consequences of colorectal anastomotic failure, or immunosuppressed individuals. Again, all facets of the operation can be achieved via minimally invasive approaches as long as the goals of the operation can be achieved in a safe fashion and physiological parameters are permitting.

Again, mention should be made of hybrid minimally invasive approaches such as the use of hand ports. These can be useful techniques particularly in the setting of more extensive inflammation and phlegmon formation. Pure laparoscopic resection is also often difficult in the setting of colovesicular fistula formation. Such approaches can minimize incision sizes and are likely to translate into decreased complications for patients. Again, the chosen operative approach is driven by the opportunity to safely achieve the goal.

In circumstances of extremis (i.e., massive resuscitation, vasopressor support), acidosis, or coagulopathy, a staged, "damage-controlled" approach is pursued. In this case source control is the only operative objective; the offending segment is resected and the afferent and efferent limb left in discontinuity, a temporary abdominal closure device is applied, and the patient is returned to the ICU for resuscitation. Recent data highlight acceptable outcomes with this approach [73].

Laparoscopic peritoneal lavage and drainage for Hinchey II and III, though briefly en vogue, have been debunked as a viable option for Hinchey III and IV diseases. In a recent randomized clinical trial comparing lavage/drainage to primary resection for acute perforated diverticulitis, lavage failed to reduce mortality or severe postoperative complications and worsened outcomes in secondary endpoints, such as need for reoperation [74]. Consideration of laparoscopically guided drainage can be considered in Hinchey I–II diseases where operative resection is not otherwise indicated, radiologic-guided percutaneous drainage is not possible, and a patient is failing to improve despite adequate antibiotic and supportive measures. There are no studies to support this approach; however, if this allows for source control, this technique may avoid definitive resection. However, as noted above, subsequent resections in patients with previous complicated disease treated with drainage are more common than in uncomplicated disease.

Take-Home Messages

1. A minimally invasive, laparoscopic approach may be safely performed in the setting of appropriate patient physiology and characteristics, independent of severity of modified Hinchey classification [27, 30, 31, 54, 55, 65].
2. Complicated diverticulitis (Hinchey Ia–II) is associated with a high risk of recurrence and subsequent complication and, thus, should prompt evaluation and preparation for elective laparoscopic colectomy with primary anastomosis [25–27].
3. Use of hand-assisted laparoscopic techniques may obviate conversion to open laparotomy yet still afford the patient many of the benefits of a total laparoscopic approach, including reduced pain, complications, and hospital length of stay [66, 75].
4. Primary anastomosis with or without proximal diversion should be considered in setting of appropriate patient physiology and tissue quality, as it is associated with reduced morbidity and mortality [71, 72].

Key References

1. Munson KD, et al. Diverticulitis. A comprehensive follow-up. Dis Colon Rectum. 1996;39(3):318–22.
2. Matrana MR, Margolin DA. Epidemiology and pathophysiology of diverticular disease. Clin Colon Rectal Surg. 2009;22(3):141–6.
3. Kozak LJ, Lees KA, DeFrances CJ. National Hospital Discharge Survey: 2003 annual summary with detailed diagnosis and procedure data. Vital Health Stat. 2006;13(160):1–206.
4. Stollman NH, Raskin JB. Diverticular disease of the colon. J Clin Gastroenterol. 1999;29(3):241–52.
5. Jacobs DO. Clinical practice. Diverticulitis. N Engl J Med. 2007;357(20):2057–66.
6. Ambrosetti P, et al. Acute left colonic diverticulitis: a prospective analysis of 226 consecutive cases. Surgery. 1994;115(5):546–50.
7. Beranbaum SL, Zausner J, Lane B. Diverticular disease of the right colon. Am J Roentgenol Radium Therapy, Nucl Med. 1972;115(2):334–48.
8. Hughes LE. Postmortem survey of diverticular disease of the colon. I. Diverticulosis and diverticulitis. Gut. 1969;10(5):336–44.
9. Bogardus ST Jr. What do we know about diverticular disease? A brief overview. J Clin Gastroenterol. 2006;40(Suppl 3):S108–11.
10. Painter NS. The aetiology of diverticulosis of the colon with special reference to the action of certain drugs on the behaviour of the colon. Ann R Coll Surg Engl. 1964;34:98–119.
11. Painter NS, et al. Segmentation and the localization of intraluminal pressure in the human colon, with special reference to the pathogenesis of colonic diverticula. Gastroenterology. 1968;54(4 Suppl):778–80.
12. Hodgson J. Effect of methylcellulose on rectal and colonic pressures in treatment of diverticular disease. Br Med J. 1972;3(5829):729–31.
13. Painter NS, Burkitt DP. Diverticular disease of the colon: a deficiency disease of western civilization. Br Med J. 1971;2(5759):450–4.
14. Hobson KG, Roberts PL. Etiology and pathophysiology of diverticular disease. Clin Colon Rectal Surg. 2004;17(3):147–53.
15. Aldoori WH, et al. A prospective study of diet and the risk of symptomatic diverticular disease in men. Am J Clin Nutr. 1994;60(5):757–64.
16. Aldoori W, Ryan-Harshman M. Preventing diverticular disease. Review of recent evidence on high-fibre diets. Can Fam Physician. 2002;48:1632–7.
17. Spiller RC. Changing views on diverticular disease: impact of aging, obesity, diet, and microbiota. Neurogastroenterol Motil. 2015;27(3):305–12.
18. Korzenik JR. Case closed? Diverticulitis: epidemiology and fiber. J Clin Gastroenterol. 2006;40(Suppl 3):S112–6.
19. Strate LL. Lifestyle factors and the course of diverticular disease. Dig Dis. 2012;30(1):35–45.
20. Wolff BG, Devine RM. Surgical management of diverticulitis. Am Surg. 2000;66(2):153–6.
21. Barat M, et al. Acute colonic diverticulitis: an update on clinical classification and management with MDCT correlation. Abdom Radiol (NY). 2016;41:1842–50.
22. Kaiser AM, et al. The management of complicated diverticulitis and the role of computed tomography. Am J Gastroenterol. 2005;100(4):910–7.
23. Kircher MF, et al. Frequency, sensitivity, and specificity of individual signs of diverticulitis on thin-section helical CT with colonic contrast material: experience with 312 cases. AJR Am J Roentgenol. 2002;178(6):1313–8.
24. Mazuski JE, et al. The surgical infection society guidelines on antimicrobial therapy for intra-abdominal infections: evidence for the recommendations. Surg Infect. 2002;3(3):175–233.
25. Devaraj B, et al. Medically treated diverticular abscess associated with high risk of recurrence and disease complications. Dis Colon Rectum. 2016;59(3):208–15.
26. Lamb MN, Kaiser AM. Elective resection versus observation after nonoperative management of complicated diverticulitis with abscess: a systematic review and meta-analysis. Dis Colon Rectum. 2014;57(12):1430–40.
27. Zapletal C, et al. Laparoscopic sigmoid resections for diverticulitis complicated by abscesses or fistulas. Int J Color Dis. 2007;22(12):1515–21.
28. Vasilevsky CA, et al. Fistulas complicating diverticulitis. Int J Color Dis. 1998;13(2):57–60.
29. Melchior S, et al. Diagnosis and surgical management of colovesical fistulas due to sigmoid diverticulitis. J Urol. 2009;182(3):978–82.
30. Cirocchi R, et al. Laparoscopic treatment of colovesical fistulas due to complicated colonic diverticular disease: a systematic review. Tech Coloproctol. 2014;18(10):873–85.
31. Bartus CM, et al. Colovesical fistula: not a contraindication to elective laparoscopic colectomy. Dis Colon Rectum. 2005;48(2):233–6.
32. Machicado GA, Jensen DM. Acute and chronic management of lower gastrointestinal bleeding: cost-effective approaches. Gastroenterologist. 1997;5(3):189–201.
33. Lewis M. And Ndsg, *Bleeding colonic diverticula*. J Clin Gastroenterol. 2008;42(10):1156–8.
34. McGuire HH Jr. Bleeding colonic diverticula. A reappraisal of natural history and management. Ann Surg. 1994;220(5):653–6.
35. Goldstein JN, et al. Four-factor prothrombin complex concentrate versus plasma for rapid vitamin K antagonist reversal in patients needing urgent surgical or invasive interventions: a phase 3b, open-label, non-inferiority, randomised trial. Lancet. 2015;385(9982):2077–87.
36. Hedges A, et al. Clinical effectiveness and safety outcomes associated with prothrombin complex concentrates. J Thromb Thrombolysis. 2016;42(1):6–10.
37. Nagata N, et al. Safety and effectiveness of early colonoscopy in Management of Acute Lower Gastrointestinal Bleeding on the basis of propensity score matching analysis. Clin Gastroenterol Hepatol. 2016;14(4):558–64.
38. Cirocchi R, et al. New trends in acute Management of Colonic Diverticular Bleeding: a systematic review. Medicine (Baltimore). 2015;94(44):e1710.
39. Jensen DM, et al. Urgent colonoscopy for the diagnosis and treatment of severe diverticular hemorrhage. N Engl J Med. 2000;342(2):78–82.
40. Navaneethan U, et al. Timing of colonoscopy and outcomes in patients with lower GI bleeding: a nationwide population-based study. Gastrointest Endosc. 2014;79(2):297–306. e12
41. Jensen DM, et al. Natural history of definitive diverticular hemorrhage based on stigmata of recent hemorrhage and colonoscopic Doppler blood flow monitoring for risk stratification and definitive hemostasis. Gastrointest Endosc. 2016;83(2):416–23.
42. Bloomfeld RS, Rockey DC, Shetzline MA. Endoscopic therapy of acute diverticular hemorrhage. Am J Gastroenterol. 2001;96(8):2367–72.
43. Kaltenbach T, et al. Colonoscopy with clipping is useful in the diagnosis and treatment of diverticular bleeding. Clin Gastroenterol Hepatol. 2012;10(2):131–7.
44. Garcia-Blazquez V, et al. Accuracy of CT angiography in the diagnosis of acute gastrointestinal bleeding: systematic review and meta-analysis. Eur Radiol. 2013;23(5):1181–90.
45. Funaki B. Endovascular intervention for the treatment of acute arterial gastrointestinal hemorrhage. Gastroenterol Clin N Am. 2002;31(3):701–13.
46. Mejaddam AY, et al. Outcomes following "rescue" superselective angioembolization for gastrointestinal hemorrhage in hemodynamically unstable patients. J Trauma Acute Care Surg. 2013;75(3):398–403.
47. Khanna A, Ognibene SJ, Koniaris LG. Embolization as first-line therapy for diverticulosis-related massive lower gastrointestinal

bleeding: evidence from a meta-analysis. J Gastrointest Surg. 2005;9(3):343–52.

48. Tan KK, Wong D, Sim R. Superselective embolization for lower gastrointestinal hemorrhage: an institutional review over 7 years. World J Surg. 2008;32(12):2707–15.

49. Kuo WT, et al. Superselective microcoil embolization for the treatment of lower gastrointestinal hemorrhage. J Vasc Interv Radiol. 2003;14(12):1503–9.

50. Broderick-Villa G, et al. Hospitalization for acute diverticulitis does not mandate routine elective colectomy. Arch Surg. 2005;140(6):576–81. discussion 581–3.

51. Salem L, et al. The timing of elective colectomy in diverticulitis: a decision analysis. J Am Coll Surg. 2004;199(6):904–12.

52. Simianu VV, et al. Number of diverticulitis episodes before resection and factors associated with earlier interventions. JAMA Surg. 2016;151(7):604–10.

53. Klarenbeek BR, et al. Laparoscopic versus open sigmoid resection for diverticular disease: follow-up assessment of the randomized control sigma trial. Surg Endosc. 2011;25(4):1121–6.

54. Gaertner WB, et al. The evolving role of laparoscopy in colonic diverticular disease: a systematic review. World J Surg. 2013;37(3):629–38.

55. Siddiqui MR, et al. Elective open versus laparoscopic sigmoid colectomy for diverticular disease: a meta-analysis with the sigma trial. World J Surg. 2010;34(12):2883–901.

56. Fleisher LA, et al. 2014 ACC/AHA guideline on perioperative cardiovascular evaluation and management of patients undergoing noncardiac surgery: a report of the American College of Cardiology/American Heart Association task force on practice guidelines. J Am Coll Cardiol. 2014;64(22):e77–137.

57. Mosquera C, Spaniolas K, Fitzgerald TL. Impact of frailty on surgical outcomes: the right patient for the right procedure. Surgery. 2016;160(2):272–80.

58. Fagard K, et al. The impact of frailty on postoperative outcomes in individuals aged 65 and over undergoing elective surgery for colorectal cancer: a systematic review. J Geriatr Oncol. 2016;7:479–91.

59. Guenaga KF, Matos D, Wille-Jorgensen P. Mechanical bowel preparation for elective colorectal surgery. Cochrane Database Syst Rev. 2011;9:CD001544.

60. Chen M, et al. Comparing mechanical bowel preparation with both oral and systemic antibiotics versus mechanical bowel preparation and systemic antibiotics alone for the prevention of surgical site infection after elective colorectal surgery: a meta-analysis of randomized controlled clinical trials. Dis Colon Rectum. 2016;59(1):70–8.

61. Nelson RL, Gladman E, Barbateskovic M. Antimicrobial prophylaxis for colorectal surgery. Cochrane Database Syst Rev. 2014;5:CD001181.

62. Darouiche RO, et al. Chlorhexidine-alcohol versus povidone-iodine for surgical-site antisepsis. N Engl J Med. 2010;362(1):18–26.

63. Fleshman JW. Laparoscopic colon and rectal surgery. In: Cameron JL, Cameron AM, editors. Current surgical therapy: expert consult. New York: Saunders; 2013. p. 1369–77.

64. Ferzli GS, Fingerhut A. Trocar placement for laparoscopic abdominal procedures: a simple standardized method. J Am Coll Surg. 2004;198(1):163–73.

65. Abedi N, McKinlay R, Park A. Laparoscopic colectomy for diverticulitis. Curr Surg. 2004;61(4):366–9.

66. Moloo H, et al. Hand assisted laparoscopic surgery versus conventional laparoscopy for colorectal surgery. Cochrane Database Syst Rev. 2010;10:CD006585.

67. Ng LW, et al. Hand-assisted laparoscopic versus total laparoscopic right colectomy: a randomized controlled trial. Color Dis. 2012;14(9):e612–7.

68. Neutzling CB, et al. Stapled versus handsewn methods for colorectal anastomosis surgery. Cochrane Database Syst Rev. 2012;2:CD003144.

69. Resegotti A, et al. Side-to-side stapled anastomosis strongly reduces anastomotic leak rates in Crohn's disease surgery. Dis Colon Rectum. 2005;48(3):464–8.

70. Choy PY, et al. Stapled versus handsewn methods for ileocolic anastomoses. Cochrane Database Syst Rev. 2011;9:CD004320.

71. Constantinides VA, et al. Primary resection with anastomosis vs. Hartmann's procedure in nonelective surgery for acute colonic diverticulitis: a systematic review. Dis Colon Rectum. 2006;49(7):966–81.

72. Salem L, Flum DR. Primary anastomosis or Hartmann's procedure for patients with diverticular peritonitis? A systematic review. Dis Colon Rectum. 2004;47(11):1953–64.

73. Kafka-Ritsch R, et al. Damage control surgery with abdominal vacuum and delayed bowel reconstruction in patients with perforated diverticulitis Hinchey III/IV. J Gastrointest Surg. 2012;16(10):1915–22.

74. Schultz JK, et al. Laparoscopic lavage vs primary resection for acute perforated diverticulitis: the SCANDIV randomized clinical trial. JAMA. 2015;314(13):1364–75.

75. Lee SW, et al. Laparoscopic vs. hand-assisted laparoscopic sigmoidectomy for diverticulitis. Dis Colon Rectum. 2006;49(4):464–9.

76. Schwesinger WH, et al. Operative management of diverticular emergencies: strategies and outcomes. Arch Surg. 2000;135(5):558–62. discussion 562–3.

Nathalie Wong-Chong and A. Sender Liberman

Minimally invasive surgery is the standard practice for many elective colorectal cases. Emergency laparoscopic colon surgery is gaining momentum and has been found to be safe and technically feasible [1]. A systematic review demonstrated earlier return of gastrointestinal function, shorter length of hospital stay, fewer complications, and lower mortality rates in those undergoing laparoscopic compared to open colectomy [2]. With advanced minimally invasive surgery expertise, management of surgical complications following colorectal surgery, such as anastomotic leak, rectal stump blowout, and small bowel volvulus, can be approached laparoscopically. The patient's hemodynamic function should be able to tolerate the physiologic effects of CO_2 pneumoperitoneum [3, 4]. Patients with abdominal compartment syndrome, poor lung compliance, bradyarrhythmias, or hemodynamic instability will not tolerate the increased intra-abdominal pressure, decreased functional residual capacity of the lung, or vagal stimulation induced by stretching of the peritoneum on insufflation that are associated with laparoscopy [4, 5]. The purpose of this chapter is to highlight the clinical and technical aspects of laparoscopic management of the common complications following colorectal surgery.

Anastomotic Leak

Failure of a colorectal anastomosis is the most feared complication of colorectal surgery. The anastomotic leak rate varies from 3% to 30% depending on risk factors and vary-

N. Wong-Chong
Department of General Surgery, McGill University Health Centre, Montreal, QC, Canada
e-mail: nathalie.wong-chong@mail.mcgill.ca

A.S. Liberman (✉)
Department of Colon & Rectal Surgery, McGill University Health Centre, Montreal, QC, Canada
e-mail: sender.liberman@mcgill.ca

ing definitions of anastomotic leak [6, 7]. It can lead to devastating consequences, including increased length of stay, increased morbidity and mortality, and reoperation [8, 9]. Early identification of anastomotic leaks is key to facilitate treatment and minimize morbidity and mortality associated with this complication.

The rate of anastomotic leak has been found to be similar or lower in laparoscopic compared to open colectomy [10, 11]. Several risk factors for anastomotic leak have been identified. In a recent meta-analysis, obesity, lower preoperative serum albumin or total protein, male sex, ongoing anticoagulation treatment, intraoperative complications, and low-volume centers were identified as independent risk factors for anastomotic leak [9]. Other risk factors include diabetes, immunosuppression, and radiation [12]. The use of perioperative nonsteroidal anti-inflammatory drugs (NSAIDS) has also been identified as a risk factor for anastomotic leak; however, the evidence for and against its use has been a controversial topic of current debate [13–15]. A nomogram created by Frasson et al. can help provide risk estimates for anastomotic leak (Fig. 13.1) [9]. This predictive model, however, is limited in the variables included.

In addition to patient factors, intraoperative and technical factors may increase the risk of anastomotic leak. The more distal the anastomosis is, the higher the risk of anastomotic failure [8]. A proper anastomosis, regardless of which method (stapled vs. hand-sewn, side to end, end to end, etc.) was used to create it, should bring together healthy, tension-free, well-perfused, and unobstructed bowel.

Intraoperative assessment of left-sided anastomoses with an air leak test can be performed via a bulb syringe and rigid or flexible endoscope. A positive test allows for immediate identification with the potential for repair, reanastomosis, or diversion. In a retrospective review of almost 1000 patients, those with positive air leak tests who were managed with intraoperative suture repair were significantly more likely to develop clinical leaks than those treated with reanastomosis or diversion [16].

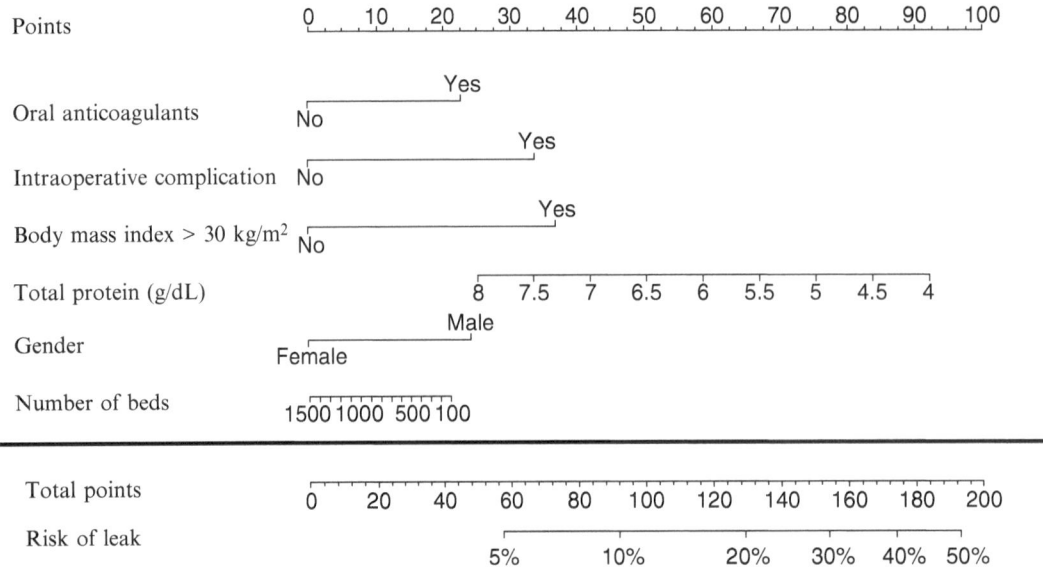

Fig. 13.1 Nomogram for prediction of expected anastomotic leak rate derived from multivariate analysis by Frasson et al. [9]. To calculate the probability of anastomotic leak, first obtain the value for each predictor by drawing a vertical line straight upward from that factor to the points' axis, then sum the points achieved for each predictor, and locate this sum on the total points' axis of the nomogram, where the probability of anastomotic leak can be located by drawing a vertical line downward

Diagnosis

Delay in recognition and intervention of an anastomotic leak is associated with increased patient morbidity and mortality [8, 9]. Clinical leaks may not always be easily identified, especially in patients who have a diverting stoma. A patient whose postoperative course veers off the standard recovery pathway should raise one's clinical suspicion of an anastomotic leak, unless otherwise proven. Routine laboratory investigations may reveal leukocytosis or increasing C-reactive protein. Postoperative tachycardia, hypotension, fever, tachypnea, oliguria, or mental status changes may occur. Worsening abdominal pain and peritonitis are less likely to occur in the absence of a large intraperitoneal leak and may be a late clinical sign.

A CT scan of the abdomen and pelvis demonstrating a large collection of free fluid, extravasation of contrast material, or a peri-anastomotic fluid collection is indicative of an anastomotic failure. Intravenous contrast may be helpful in identifying rim-enhancing abscesses, while carefully administered rectal contrast can be useful in evaluating a colorectal anastomosis. Flexible or rigid endoscopy may provide additional information regarding the exact location and extent of anastomotic dehiscence.

Management

The management of anastomotic failure depends on the patient's clinical status, as some leaks are asymptomatic and others can result in sepsis and septic shock, mandating prompt surgical management.

The incidence of anastomotic leakage varies considerably among published clinical data in part owing to the lack of a standardized definition of this complication. The International Study Group of Rectal Cancer proposed a grading system for the management of colorectal anastomotic leaks (Fig. 13.2) [17]. Grade A leaks can be managed expectantly. Broad-spectrum antibiotics may be indicated depending on the clinical scenario. These leaks occur in patients who are asymptomatic or minimally symptomatic. Grade A leaks are identified by radiographic findings of a peri-anastomotic fluid collection, leakage of contrast through the anastomosis, or observation of new drainage of enteric contents through either a drain or through a fistula. Although this mild form of anastomotic leakage does not require active intervention, closure of a diverting ileostomy/colostomy should be delayed until the leak has resolved.

Patients with Grade B leaks are clinically symptomatic. Grade B leaks require therapeutic intervention, but not necessarily reoperation. These leaks usually delay hospital discharge; however, these patients may have a relatively normal postoperative course, especially in the era of enhanced recovery after surgery (ERAS) programs where patients are staying in hospital for shorter periods of time. As such, a significant portion of Grade B leaks present as readmissions owing to the late development of symptoms. Treatment is usually with broad-spectrum antibiotics and percutaneous, transvaginal, or transanal drainage of fluid collections.

Grade A and Grade B leaks that fail conservative therapy may become upgraded to Grade C, defined as anastomotic leaks requiring urgent re-exploration. Surgical treatment is performed with the goal of controlling life-threatening sepsis.

Proposal for the definition and severity grading of anastomotic leakage after anterior resection of the rectum

Definition		Defect of the intestinal wall integrity at the colorectel or colo-anal anastomotic site (including suture and staple lines of neorectal reservoirs) leading to a communication between the intra-and extraluminal compartments. A pelvic abscess close to the anastomosis is also considered as anastomotic leakage.
Grade	A	Anastomotic leakage requiring no active therapeutic intervention
	B	Anastomotic leakage requiring active therapeutic intervention but manageable without re-laparotomy
	C	Anastomotic leakage requiring re-laparotomy

Fig. 13.2 Grading system for the management of colorectal anastomotic leaks by the International Study Group of Rectal Cancer [17]

Management may range from washout with drain placement and diverting loop ileostomy to taking down the anastomosis with end colostomy. Retrospective analysis of laparoscopic peritoneal lavage and ileostomy creation has shown low morbidity and mortality rates compared with open surgery [18].

A laparoscopic approach may be feasible based on the patient's surgical history and clinical status. A clinically unstable patient with generalized peritonitis should be managed as expediently as possible, without further metabolic derangement that can occur with insufflation of the abdominal cavity with carbon dioxide. As such, laparoscopy should not be attempted. However, in patients who can clinically tolerate laparoscopy, the decision to reoperate from a minimally invasive approach depends on the initial operative approach, the timing from the last surgery, and the risk of complications including adhesiolysis and iatrogenic injury.

Patients selected for laparoscopic evaluation should be positioned supine (split-leg or modified lithotomy to provide access to the rectum, as necessary). The arms should be tucked to the patient's side and the patient secured to the table to allow for tilting in different vectors for appropriate washout and repair/resection. We recommend an open Hasson technique with direct visualization to enter the abdomen laparoscopically. A laparoscopic camera can then be inserted to survey the abdomen and determine whether intra-abdominal conditions are favorable or hostile to proceed laparoscopically. Trocars should be placed as appropriate for the procedure planned, recognizing the need for additional assistant ports to allow for adequate visualization, irrigation, and drainage. Poor intraoperative exposure and progress due to dilated loops of bowel, intra-abdominal adhesions, inadequate washout, or clinical deterioration should prompt conversion to laparotomy.

Depending on the level of the anastomosis, decisions regarding repair vs. diversion vs. takedown and end stoma must be made. Repairing a leak requires adequate visualization of the problem. For example, an ileoileal or ileocolic anastomosis may be freshened up and repaired if detected early, or it may need to be resected and reanastomosed. This can be done fully laparoscopically, or the involved segment can be exteriorized for the repair. The extraction site of the initial surgery would be the extraction site of preference in

order to avoid creating separate incisions unnecessarily, but this may not always be possible.

For a rectal anastomosis, it is generally best to not take down the anastomosis, as it is not possible to reanastomose in the context of intra-abdominal sepsis. The authors would advise performing a lavage, leaving a drain in the pelvis and diverting proximally. If the leak is small, it will often heal, eliminating the need for further rectal repair. If the leak doesn't heal, any future intervention will be easier to perform if the proximal bowel is still in place, helping to prevent retraction of the rectum behind the bladder, prostate, or vagina. If the anastomotic disruption is major or complete, we would generally take down the anastomosis and create an end colostomy. Closing the rectal stump may not be possible laparoscopically, but if there is any way to suture or staple it closed, it would help prevent ongoing contamination. Again, this may be attempted laparoscopically, but if not possible, a low midline of Pfannenstiel incision may be required.

Postoperative care is similar to other causes of intra-abdominal sepsis. Patients managed laparoscopically may report shoulder/back pain referred from the diaphragm, which should resolve within 24–48 h. Similarly, CO_2 pneumoperitoneum from laparoscopic surgery may be present on chest radiographs done in the postanesthetic care unit or the intensive care unit postoperatively but should resolved within 24–48 h. Ongoing abdominal or back pain associated with lack of clinical improvement or clinical deterioration should prompt further investigations into ongoing anastomotic leak or other postoperative complications.

Novel techniques such as self-expanding metal stents or covered stents are still in experimental phases. Issues and concerns with stent migration have limited the clinical adoption of this intervention.

Rectal Stump Leak

Despite recent trials analyzing the role for laparoscopic lavage or resection and anastomosis for diverticulitis, the Hartmann's procedure is still commonly performed for perforated feculent diverticulitis, as well as for emergency cases of sigmoid volvulus, trauma, perforated sigmoid cancer, and acute colitis. Although the rates are declining, subtotal colectomy with an end ileostomy continues to be the mainstay of surgical therapy for acute fulminant colitis, such as for ulcerative colitis, ischemic colitis, or *C. difficile* colitis [19]. These operations leave patients with a rectal stump that has either a staple or suture line that is at risk of leakage. The rate of rectal stump leak for diverticulitis is not well documented in the literature. Following subtotal colectomy for acute colitis, the risk of rectal stump leak resulting in pelvic sepsis ranges from 4% to 12% (Table 13.1) [20–27]. The rate is highest for short intrapelvic stumps (33%) compared to intraperitoneal (6–12%) and subcutaneous (3–4%) rectal stumps [21–24, 26]. A recent review of the American College of Surgeons National Surgical Quality Improvement Program databases from 2012 to 2015 reported a 4.1% rectal stump leak rate (96 of 2349 patients) [28]. Longer operative time and contaminated wounds were associated with rectal stump leaks. The study found that rectal stump leak was a significant predictor of mortality within 30 days of surgery (OR 3.608 (95% CI 1.515–8.594)), reoperation (OR 7.319 (95% CI 41.5–12.908)), readmission (OR 5.762 (95%CI 4.316–9.718)), and postoperative ileus (OR 2.116 (95%CI 1.27–3.527)).

Diagnosis

A rectal stump leak (Fig. 13.3) should be suspected in patients with signs and symptoms of pelvic sepsis, persistent or worsening abdominal pain, fever, leukocytosis, prolonged postoperative ileus, and nausea/vomiting. In a review of eleven cases by Schien et al., four were associated with small

bowel fistula and eight with abdominal wall dehiscence [29]. When suspected, an abdominal/pelvic CT scan can confirm the diagnosis. Extra-luminal air or fluid may be seen above the rectal stump or elsewhere in the peritoneal cavity, which may be associated with a localized collection.

Management

Patients with peritonitis or signs of sepsis should have emergency surgery. Clinically stable patients without generalized peritonitis and with CT evidence of localized collections without any free fluid or air may be managed with CT or ultrasound-guided percutaneous drainage. Broad-spectrum antibiotics should be initiated promptly.

Patients selected for laparoscopic operative management should be positioned supine with the arms tucked to the patient's side. Legs should be positioned in a split-leg or modified lithotomy position. Similar to other reoperative cases, entry to the abdomen should be obtained via an open Hasson technique that allows for direct visualization to reduce the risk of injury upon entry. These patients often have a postoperative ileus, and as such the Veress needle should be avoided due to the presence of dilated loops of bowel or a distended stomach. Trocars may be placed through the previous port sites (Fig. 13.4), usually a 5 or 12 mm port in the right lower quadrant two fingerbreadths superior and medial to the anterior superior iliac spine and a 5 mm port in the right upper quadrant. An additional 5 mm assistant port can be inserted near the epigastrium or in the left lower quadrant. The abdomen and pelvis are then assessed. Purulent/

Table 13.1 Reports on (colo)rectal stump-related complications following total abdominal colectomy for ulcerative colitis

Authors	Year	Indications for surgery	Timing of surgery	Location of defunctionalized stump	Patient number	Pelvic abscess rate, %	Wound infection rate, %
Carter et al. [6]	1991	Acute ulcerative colitis	N/A	Subcutaneous	55	4	13
				Intraperitoneal	51	12	0
Kyle et al. [7]	1992	Fulminant colitis, megacolon	Emergent/urgent	Intraperitoneal	23	8	4
Ng et al. [8]	1992	Acute colitis, megacolon, perforation	Emergent	Subcutaneous	32	3	6
McKee et al. [9]	1995	Acute colitis, megacolon, perforation	Mixed[a]	Intraperitoneal	62	6	0
Wojdemann et al. [10]	1995	Acute colitis, megacolon, perforation	Emergent	Intraperitoneal	147	3	8
Karch et al. [11]	1995	IBD colitis	N/A	Intraperitoneal	114	3	N/A
Trickett et al. [12]	2005	Acute colitis, megacolon, perforation	Emergent	Subcutaneous	10	0	30
				Intraperitoneal	27	7	26
Gu (current study)	2012	Severe colitis	Mixed[b]	Subcutaneous	105	4	13
				Intraperitoneal	99	6	5

N/A not available

[a]Composed of emergent surgery in 60%, urgent surgery in 35%, and elective surgery in 5% of cases

[b]Composed of emergent surgery in 15%, urgent surgery in 40%, and elective surgery in 45% of cases

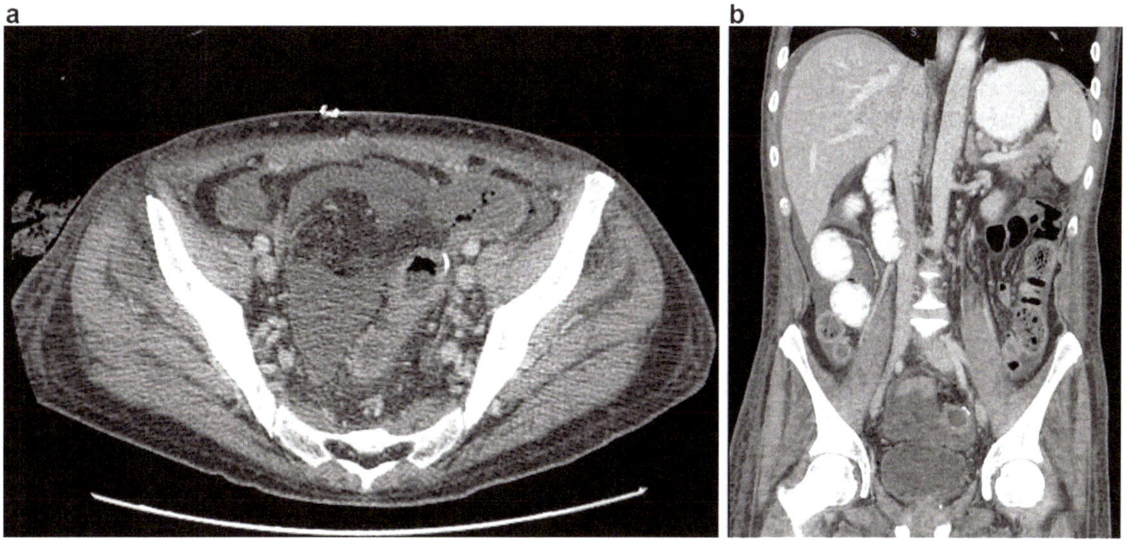

a

b

Fig. 13.3 (**a**, **b**) Rectal stump leak. Pelvic collection adjacent to rectal stump

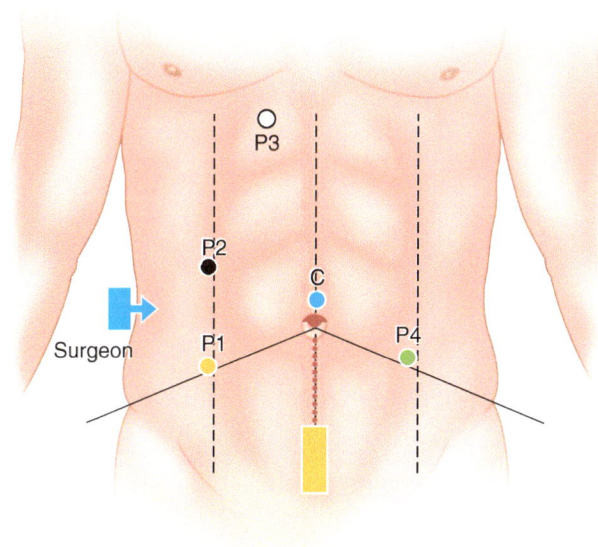

Fig. 13.4 Port placement

feculent fluid is washed out, and the abdomen is irrigated with warmed saline.

The management of a rectal stump blowout or leak is controversial. One option is to bring the end up as a mucous fistula. However, this is not an option for shorter rectal stumps that do not reach the abdominal wall. The second option is to debride and close the stump and leave it in the subcutaneous place at the lower end of a midline wound. This option also requires a long rectal stump and carries the risk of complications associated with retained inflamed bowel if the indication for surgery was colitis. The third option is to washout and

debride any devitalized tissue and leave the rectum open. A rectal tube can be inserted into the top of the rectal stump, secured to the rectum with a purse string suture, and brought out through the abdominal wall. This functions as a pseudo-mucous fistula for short rectal stumps. A fourth option is to debride and reclose the rectal stump; however, restapling or suturing a short and retracted stump can lead to recurrent breakdown [29]. Regardless of the management of the top of the rectal stump, it is critical that all fecal material should be removed and irrigated from the rectum and pelvis. A rectal tube can be inserted transanally and secured to the perianal skin. In addition, a sump drain can be placed in the pelvis, especially when there is concern for ongoing contamination or incomplete evacuation of infected debris.

Reopening the previous extraction site (lower midline or Pfannenstiel) may facilitate the creation of a mucous fistula or secure the purse string.

An open approach should be used in patients unable to tolerate laparoscopy. Hemodynamic instability, uncontrollable bleeding, and iatrogenic injuries to surrounding organs (e.g., ureter, small bowel) are indications for converting from a laparoscopic to open technique. As in all cases of fecal or purulent peritonitis, a second look may be advised if the patient's clinical condition warrants it in the following 24–48 h. We would advise closing the fascia completely instead of placing temporary abdominal closures to prevent retraction of the fascia.

Ileal J-Pouch Volvulus

An ileal pouch-anal anastomosis (IPAA) allows restoration of fecal continence in select patients who have undergone a total proctocolectomy for ulcerative colitis or familial adenomatous polyposis (FAP). Well-known complications following

IPAA include pouchitis, anastomotic leak, and small bowel obstruction. J-pouch volvulus leading to obstruction is exceedingly rare. There are only a few case reports in the literature [30–34]. Most cases occur many years after pouch creation. J-pouch volvulus may result in pouch necrosis if diagnosis and/or surgical treatment is delayed.

Diagnosis

A careful history, including a surgical history of a total proctocolectomy and IPAA, should be elicited. Clinical symptoms of J-pouch volvulus include colicky pain, fever, and vomiting. On examination, there may be evidence of abdominal distension, generalized abdominal tenderness, and features suggestive of small bowel obstruction. An abdominal CT scan with intravenous and oral contrast may demonstrate a dilated proximal small bowel with a transition point in the distal ileum. Mesenteric swirling and signs of intestinal ischemia may also be present. If clinically stable, flexible

pouchoscopy can be used to evaluate the mucosa for viability and for endoscopic decompression [33].

We recently had a 20-year-old male patient with ulcerative colitis who underwent a two-staged IPAA procedure for failure of medical management (laparoscopic total abdominal colectomy with end ileostomy, followed by completion proctectomy and IPAA 6 months later). Two months after IPAA creation, he presented with intermittent abdominal pain, occurring several times a day, seemingly unrelated to meals. He was having 6–8 bowel movements a day, not uncommon following pouch surgery. An abdominal CT scan revealed mesenteric swirling and dilated loops of small bowel with no evidence of intestinal ischemia (Fig. 13.5).

Management

Following fluid resuscitation and nasogastric decompression, emergency surgery should be performed to prevent pouch ischemia and necrosis. A laparoscopic approach can

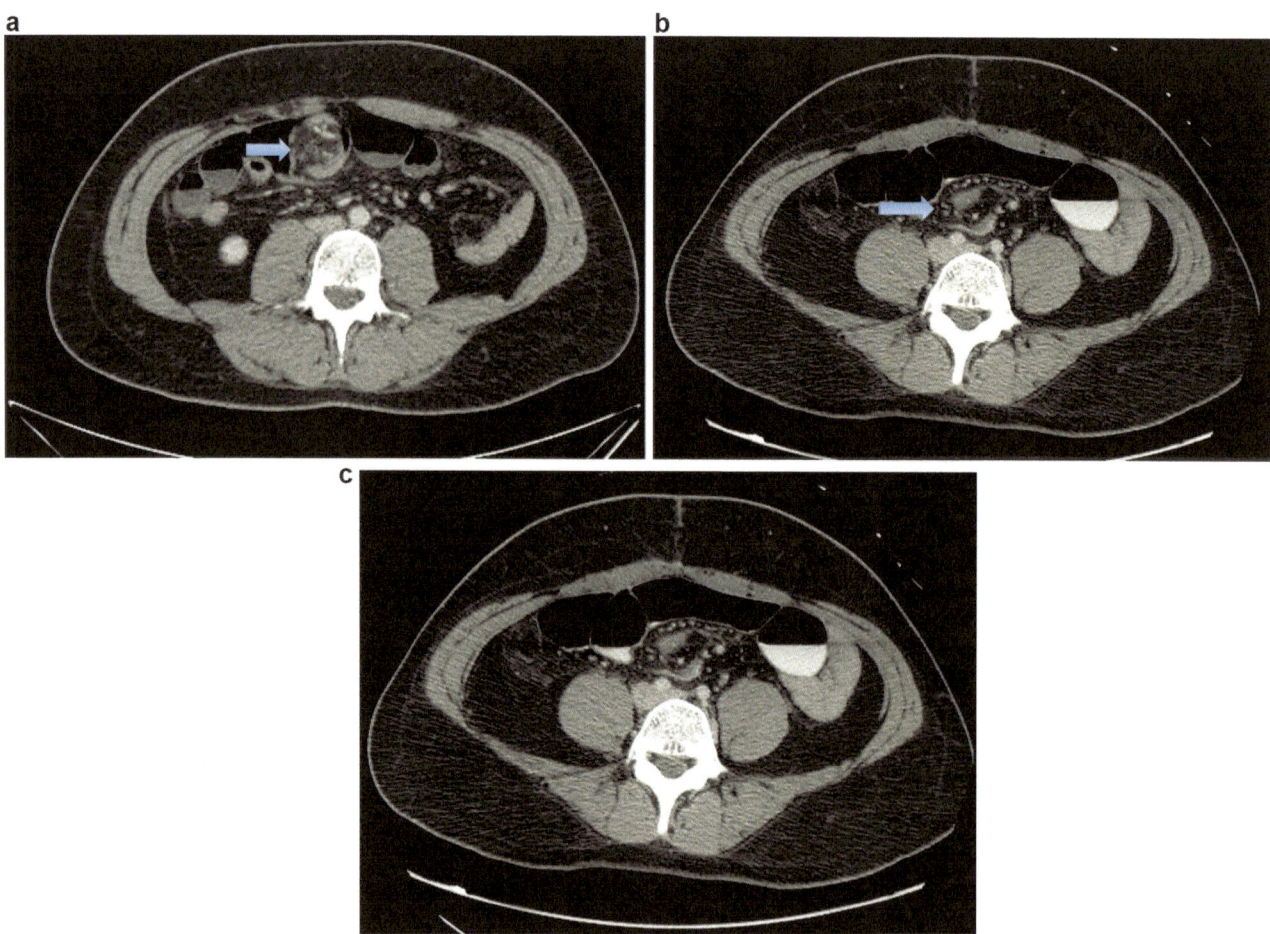

Fig. 13.5 (**a–c**) CT abdomen of patient presenting with nausea and vomiting post-total proctocolectomy and IPAA. Characteristic findings of J-pouch volvulus: dilated loops of small bowel with air-fluid levels and mesenteric swirling (*arrows*)

be used via a Hasson technique if sufficient gastrointestinal decompression can be obtained via nasogastric tube or flexible sigmoidoscopy. However, if the abdomen is severely distended leaving no domain for pneumoperitoneum, conversion to laparotomy is indicated.

If it is safe to proceed laparoscopically, two 5 mm trocars can be placed in the left abdomen, one in the left lower quadrant, and one in the left upper quadrant. The orientation and viability of the bowel can then be examined using two atraumatic bowel graspers. If the diagnosis of small bowel volvulus is confirmed and there is no evidence of necrosis, the bowel can be carefully untwisted. Care must be taken to avoid injury to the intestines as even atraumatic graspers can cause damage to severely dilated bowel. After untwisting the bowel, the pouch can be deflated using a transanal catheter or flexible endoscopy, and both the pouch and remainder of the bowel should be run in its entirety to determine viability.

If the pouch is viable, pouch pexy can be performed using sutures placed either to the left side of the anterior abdominal wall or to the retroperitoneum. Pouch excision is warranted

of it appears to be irreversibly ischemic [35]. Gangrenous bowel is excised and an end ileostomy is fashioned. In the case of small bowel volvulus around the mesenteric axis, the peritoneum of the mesenteric can be sutured to the retroperitoneum using a 2.0 silk suture.

With our case patient, the abdomen was too distended to proceed laparoscopically. We performed a lower midline laparotomy. The small bowel was chronically distended to over 5 cm. There were virtually no intra-abdominal adhesions. He had developed an internal hernia with small bowel volvulus around the mesentery secondary to an omental adhesion causing an obstruction to his pouch above the ileal-anal anastomosis (Fig. 13.6). The omental band was lysed. The bowel was detorted, and the mesenteric defect was sutured to the retroperitoneum using 2.0 silk. Pouchoscopy revealed chronic edema and ulcerated mucosa at the level of obstruction from the omental adhesion. The rest of the pouch was intact, including the staple line. In light of these findings, a diverting ileostomy was created. Postoperatively he had a prolonged ileus but recovered well.

Fig. 13.6 (a–c) Intraoperative findings of small bowel and J-pouch volvulus (**a**) chronically dilated loops of the small bowel with loop of the small intestine under the mesentery (*arrow*). (**b**) Bowel exteriorized with arrow demonstrating distended pouch and bowel loops herniating under small bowel mesentery. (**c**) Bowel untwisted and mesenteric peritoneum sutured to the retroperitoneum (*arrow*)

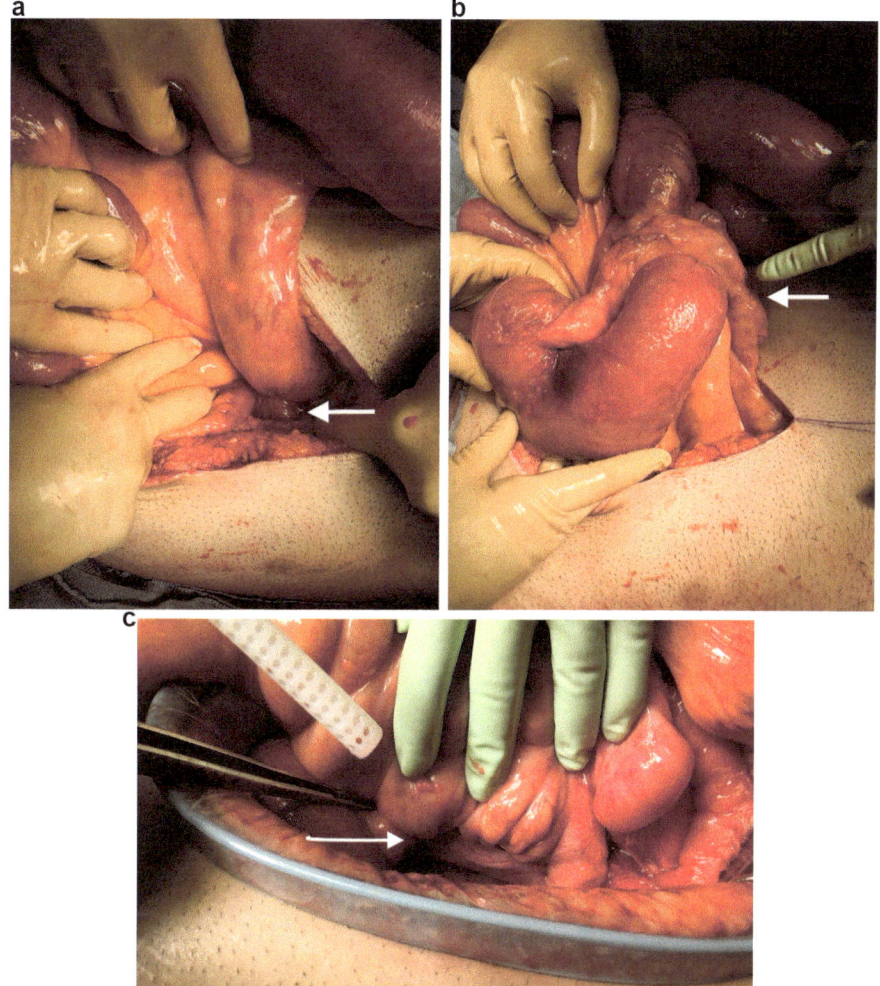

Postoperative care is similar to other causes of small bowel obstruction or volvulus. Diet should be advanced once intestinal function resumes.

There is no evidence to suggest preventative pouch pexy during the primary pouch surgery to prevent volvulus. However, given the rare occurrence of this complication and the possible complications due to pouch pexy, such as an internal hernia, routine application of pouch pexy may not be justified.

Conclusion

Complications from colorectal surgery, such as anastomotic leak, rectal stump blowout, or pouch volvulus, can be safely managed laparoscopically in the appropriate clinical scenario. Laparoscopic management has been associated with decreased length of stay and earlier return of gastrointestinal function [2]. The patient should be clinically stable and able to tolerate pneumoperitoneum. The surgeon should have surgical expertise in minimally invasive surgery. Intra-abdominal adhesions, severe bowel distension, or inadequate visualization that cannot be optimized with laparoscopic takedown, nasogastric decompression, or additional ports may require conversion to laparotomy. However, even performing part of the operation laparoscopically can minimize the size of the incision and/or the extent of the dissection when conversion to open surgery is required.

Take-Home Messages

1. Complications following colorectal surgery can be managed laparoscopically in the appropriate patient and clinical scenario.
2. Positioning the patient in the split-leg or modified lithotomy position will provide access to the rectum, allowing for intraoperative DRE, staplers, or endoscopy/proctoscopy.
3. The abdomen should be entered under direct visualization using a Hasson technique. The Veress needle approach should be avoided in re-explorative surgery due to risk of adhesions or distended bowel, which may lead to iatrogenic injury.
4. Anastomotic leaks, rectal stump blowout, and J-pouch volvulus can be managed laparoscopically using the same clinical principals and judgment applicable to open surgery.
5. A limited lower midline or Pfannenstiel incision can be used for specimen extraction, to facilitate stapling or to gain access to the rectal stump.

Key References

1. Titu LV, Zafar N, Phillips SM, Greenslade GL, Dixon AR. Emergency laparoscopic surgery for complicated diverticular disease. Color Dis. 2009;11(4):401–4.
2. Harji DP, Griffiths B, Burke D, Sagar PM. Systematic review of emergency laparoscopic colorectal resection. Br J Surg. 2014;101(1):e126–33.
3. McLaughlin JG, Scheeres DE, Dean RJ, Bonnell BW. The adverse hemodynamic effects of laparoscopic cholecystectomy. Surg Endosc. 1995;9(2):121–4.
4. Dexter SP, Vucevic M, Gibson J, McMahon MJ. Hemodynamic consequences of high- and low-pressure capnoperitoneum during laparoscopic cholecystectomy. Surg Endosc. 1999;13(4):376–81.
5. Myles PS. Bradyarrhythmias and laparoscopy: a prospective study of heart rate changes with laparoscopy. Aust N Z J Obstet Gynaecol. 1991;31(2):171–3.
6. Kingham TP, Pachter HL. Colonic anastomotic leak: risk factors, diagnosis, and treatment. J Am Coll Surg. 2009;208(2):269–78.
7. Peel AL, Taylor EW. Proposed definitions for the audit of postoperative infection: a discussion paper. Surgical Infection Study Group. Ann R Coll Surg Engl. 1991;73(6):385–8.
8. Mirnezami A, Mirnezami R, Chandrakumaran K, Sasapu K, Sagar P, Finan P. Increased local recurrence and reduced survival from colorectal cancer following anastomotic leak: systematic review and meta-analysis. Ann Surg. 2011;253(5):890–9.
9. Frasson M, Flor-Lorente B, Rodriguez JL, et al. Risk factors for anastomotic leak after colon resection for cancer: multivariate analysis and nomogram from a multicentric, prospective, National Study with 3193 patients. Ann Surg. 2015;262(2):321–30.
10. Murray AC, Chiuzan C, Kiran RP. Risk of anastomotic leak after laparoscopic versus open colectomy. Surg Endosc. 2016;30(12):5275–82.
11. van der Pas MH, Haglind E, Cuesta MA, et al. Laparoscopic versus open surgery for rectal cancer (COLOR II): short-term outcomes of a randomised, phase 3 trial. Lancet Oncol. 2013;14(3):210–8.
12. Thomas MS, Margolin DA. Management of colorectal anastomotic leak. Clin Colon Rectal Surg. 2016;29(2):138–44.
13. Bhangu A, Singh P, Fitzgerald JE, Slesser A, Tekkis P. Postoperative nonsteroidal anti-inflammatory drugs and risk of anastomotic leak: meta-analysis of clinical and experimental studies. World J Surg. 2014;38(9):2247–57.
14. Van Koughnett JA, Wexner SD. Surgery. NSAIDs and risk of anastomotic leaks after colorectal surgery. Nat Rev Gastroenterol Hepatol. 2014;11(9):523–4.
15. Rutegard M, Westermark S, Kverneng Hultberg D, Haapamaki M, Matthiessen P, Rutegard J. Non-steroidal anti-inflammatory drug use and risk of anastomotic leakage after anterior resection: a protocol-based study. Dig Surg. 2016;33(2):129–35.
16. Ricciardi R, Roberts PL, Marcello PW, Hall JF, Read TE, Schoetz DJ. Anastomotic leak testing after colorectal resection: what are the data? Arch Surg. 2009;144(5):407–11. discussion 411–402.
17. Rahbari NN, Weitz J, Hohenberger W, et al. Definition and grading of anastomotic leakage following anterior resection of the rectum: a proposal by the International Study Group of Rectal Cancer. Surgery. 2010;147(3):339–51.
18. Lee CM, Huh JW, Yun SH, et al. Laparoscopic versus open reintervention for anastomotic leakage following minimally invasive colorectal surgery. Surg Endosc. 2015;29(4):931–6.
19. Annese V, Duricova D, Gower-Rousseau C, Jess T, Langholz E. Impact of new treatments on hospitalisation, surgery, infection, and mortality in IBD: a focus paper by the epidemiology committee of ECCO. J Crohns Colitis. 2016;10(2):216–25.

20. Gu J, Stocchi L, Remzi F, Kiran RP. Intraperitoneal or subcutaneous: does location of the (colo)rectal stump influence outcomes after laparoscopic total abdominal colectomy for ulcerative colitis? Dis Colon Rectum. 2013;56(5):615–21.
21. Carter FM, McLeod RS, Cohen Z. Subtotal colectomy for ulcerative colitis: complications related to the rectal remnant. Dis Colon Rectum. 1991;34(11):1005–9.
22. Kyle SM, Steyn RS, Keenan RA. Management of the rectum following colectomy for acute colitis. Aust N Z J Surg. 1992;62(3):196–9.
23. Wojdemann M, Wettergren A, Hartvigsen A, Myrhoj T, Svendsen LB, Bulow S. Closure of rectal stump after colectomy for acute colitis. Int J Color Dis. 1995;10(4):197–9.
24. McKee RF, Keenan RA, Munro A. Colectomy for acute colitis: is it safe to close the rectal stump? Int J Color Dis. 1995;10(4):222–4.
25. Trickett JP, Tilney HS, Gudgeon AM, Mellor SG, Edwards DP. Management of the rectal stump after emergency sub-total colectomy: which surgical option is associated with the lowest morbidity? Color Dis. 2005;7(5):519–22.
26. Ng RL, Davies AH, Grace RH, Mortensen NJ. Subcutaneous rectal stump closure after emergency subtotal colectomy. Br J Surg. 1992;79(7):701–3.
27. Karch LA, Bauer JJ, Gorfine SR, Gelernt IM. Subtotal colectomy with Hartmann's pouch for inflammatory bowel disease. Dis Colon Rectum. 1995;38(6):635–9.
28. Dan AVCAM N., Faria J., Gordon P., Boutros M. Distal stump leaks following a Hartmann's procedure: an ACS-NSQIP study of risks and outcomes [ABSTRACT]. ASCRS 2017 Annual Scientific Meeting. 2017.
29. Schein M, Kopelman D, Nitecki S, Hashmonai M. Management of the leaking rectal stump after Hartmann's procedure. Am J Surg. 1993;165(2):285–7.
30. Mullen MG, Cullen JM, Michaels AD, Hedrick TL, Friel CM. Ileal j-pouch volvulus following total proctocolectomy for ulcerative colitis. J Gastrointest Surg. 2016;20(5):1072–3.
31. Patel S, Salotera G, Gurjar S, Hewes J, Ahmed I, Andrews B. Ileo-anal pouch necrosis secondary to small bowel volvulus: a case report. World J Emerg Surg. 2008;3:18.
32. Catalano O. Small bowel volvulus following ileal pouch-anal anastomosis: CT demonstration. Eur J Radiol. 1996;23(2):115–7.
33. Warren C, O'Donnell ME, Gardiner KR, Irwin T. Successful management of ileo-anal pouch volvulus. Color Dis. 2011;13(1):106–7.
34. Arima K, Watanabe M, Iwatsuki M, et al. Volvulus of an ileal pouch-rectal anastomosis after subtotal colectomy for ulcerative colitis: report of a case. Surg Today. 2014;44(12):2382–4.
35. Sherman J, Greenstein AJ, Greenstein AJ. Ileal j pouch complications and surgical solutions: a review. Inflamm Bowel Dis. 2014;20(9):1678–85.

Paul Waltz and Brian S. Zuckerbraun

Introduction

Clostridium difficile is a gram-positive, spore-forming bacillus that was discovered in the mid-1970s to be the cause of antibiotic or clindamycin-induced diarrheal illness. It has since become increasingly recognized that many different classes of antibiotics can promote a change in the gut microbiome that can lead to colonization and/or overgrowth of C. difficile within the colon, leading to infection and the diarrheal illness [1]. The temporal aspect in relationship to antibiotic exposure is usually within 2 weeks; however, the Center for Disease Control definition and presumed causality extends the associated risk period up to 3 months. Other risk factors associated with infection include changing gastric pH with pharmacological antacids, lack of an enteral diet, gastrointestinal surgery, hospitalization or institutionalization, and advanced age. These factors can be explained by decreased or altered host defenses, changes in normal microbiome, and increased environmental exposures.

The pathophysiology of infection after colonization is increased proliferation and overgrowth of C. difficile. Importantly, the clinical disease only occurs with toxin producing strains. Two toxins, toxin A and toxin B, are generally thought to be responsible for the development of the clinical syndrome. These toxins result in an inflammatory response, alterations in colonocyte cytoskeletal structure and tight junctions, and apoptosis leading to the clinical symptoms of diarrhea. Animal models reveal that toxin B may be the more potent of the two toxins, with toxin A inducing more focal effects [2].

Approximately a decade ago, the discovery of a somewhat common but hypervirulent strain was made. Termed the BI/NAP1/ ribotype 027, this strain is associated with higher levels of toxin production due to a mutation in the regulatory gene tcdC. Recent reports from Australia detailing another hypervirulent strain (ribotype 244) with high associated disease severity and mortality raises even more concern about the ever-changing microbiology which can greatly impact disease severity, treatment, and outcomes [3].

Disease Severity and Medical Therapy

The clinical syndrome of CDI is almost always associated with watery, foul smelling diarrhea with mild abdominal pain and cramping (Table 14.1). Abdominal distention may be present and a concerning sign of worsening disease if associated with the development of ileus, which may be indicated by an abrupt lack of diarrhea, with continued abdominal pain and systemic symptoms. Tachycardia and hypotension can be present in all patients if diarrhea is significant enough to cause volume depletion, but these signs are typically reflective of an increasing severity of disease and worsening systemic illness. This is also true of the presence of fever. Patients often have associated increased serum white blood cell counts. Other common lab abnormalities will include elevated creatinine.

It is important to accurately stage the severity of disease to ensure treatment is appropriately escalated and patients at higher risk of clinical deterioration are identified early. Though several severity staging criteria have been proposed, the recent criteria proposed by the American College of Gastroenterology (ACG) is relatively simple and attempts to define clear criteria to identify patients of concern for failure of medical therapy and clinical deterioration [4]. Patients are stratified into mild, moderate, severe, and sever complicated

P. Waltz
Department of Surgery, University of Pittsburgh Medical Center, Pittsburgh, PA, USA

B.S. Zuckerbraun (✉)
University of Pittsburgh Medical Center, VA Pittsburgh Healthcare System, Pittsburgh, PA, USA
e-mail: zuckerbraunbs@upmc.edu

© Springer International Publishing AG 2018
K.A. Khwaja, J.J. Diaz (eds.), *Minimally Invasive Acute Care Surgery*, https://doi.org/10.1007/978-3-319-64723-4_14

(Table 14.2). Criteria used to define severe disease include a serum white blood cell count greater than or equal to 15,000, a serum albumin less than 3.0 g/dL, and abdominal pain. Patients qualify as severe if they have at least two of these criteria. While these criteria are not specific, they were chosen based upon the association of increased risk of mortality and need for operative intervention. Higher white count may occur with increasing levels of toxin production. Lower albumin may suggest some degree of malnutrition or be an acute change in critical illness, both of which are likely risk factors for poor outcomes.

Several scoring systems have attempted to specifically help clinicians determine failure of medical therapy or the need for operation. These scores use a combination of expert consensus or multivariate analyses. These scores are highlighted and compared in Table 14.3.

The initial treatment of patients with CDI should follow the same basic principles. Patients with volume depletion should receive adequate fluid resuscitation and electrolyte repletion. A regular diet should be continued in patients if there is no contraindication. This helps promote normal colonic flora and colonocyte health. Antimotility agents should be avoided. Systemic antibiotics for other indications should be discontinued if possible. If not possible, and CDI

developed while on the current antibiotic regimen, a new antibiotic regimen should be chosen avoiding clindamycin, second and third generation cephalosporins, and fluoroquinolones.

The choice of antibiotics for the treatment of CDI is based upon the severity. Most suggested regimens use metronidazole 500 mg oral/enteral three times a day for mild or moderate disease. If a patient is NPO, then the intravenous form is acceptable and will reach effective colonic concentrations during the diarrheal state via hepatic excretion. Vancomycin has been the most commonly advocated therapy for severe disease. The usual dose is 125 mg oral/enteral four times per day. Vancomycin is not effective in the intravenous form. In patients with severe complicated disease, a combination of intravenous metronidazole plus vancomycin orally/enterally has been advocated. While there is a lack of convincing evidence, an increased vancomycin dose of 500 mg oral/enteral four times daily can be considered in severe cases. This "belt and suspenders" approach is chosen given the overall poor prognosis of these patients and the difficulty in predicting progression of disease. Vancomycin enemas also have a role in the treatment of patients with ileus or distention and are discussed further below.

Fidaxomicin, a macrocyclic antibiotic approved in 2011 for the treatment of CDI, has been shown to be non-inferior to vancomycin for initial cure with studies suggesting a lower recurrence rate [5]. At this point, fidaxomicin seems to be finding a niche in the setting of recurrent disease.

Recurrence of infection occurs in up to approximately 25% of patients, and in those who recur, subsequent recurrences happen with even increasing incidences. Multiple regimens have been proposed in the setting of recurrences. First recurrences should be treated with vancomycin. It is often recommended that second recurrences are treated with

Table 14.1 Signs/symptoms of CDI

Sign/symptom	Frequency (%)
Diarrhea	99
Leukocytosis	50
Bandemia	50
Abdominal pain	32
Fever	28
Hypoalbuminemia	15

Table 14.2 CDI severity scoring system and summary of recommended treatments

Severity	Criteria	Treatment
Mild	Diarrhea	Metronidazole 500 mg PO tid
Moderate	Diarrhea plus any additional signs or symptoms not meeting severe or complicated criteria	Metronidazole 500 mg PO tid

Severe	Any two of the following:
	    WBC $\geq$ 15,000 cells/mm^3,
	    Serum albumin <3 g/dL
	    Abdominal tenderness
		Vancomycin 125 mg PO qid

Complicated	Any one of the following:
	    Admission to intensive care unit for CDI
	    Hypotension with or without required use of vasopressors
	    Fever $\geq$38.5°
	    Ileus or significant abdominal distention
	    Mental status changes
	    WBC $\geq$ 35,000 cells/mm^3
	    Serum lactate levels greater than 2.2 mmol/Liter
	    End organ failure (mechanical ventilation, renal failure, etc.)
		Metronidazole 500 mg IV tid
		+
		Vancomycin 125 mg PO qid
		+
		Vancomycin 500 mg in 500 mL saline as enema qid (if ileus or distended)
		+
		Surgical consultation

Adapted from Guidelines of the American College of Gastroenterology [4]

Table 14.3 Comparison of C. difficile scoring systems

Score	Criteria (pts)	Comments
UPMC score [10, 15]	Immunosuppression and/or chronic medical condition (1 pt) Abdominal pain or distention (1 pt) Hypoalbuminemia (<3 g/dl) (1 pt) Fever >38.5 (1 pt) ICU admission (1 pt) CT scan with pancolitis (2 pts) WBC > 15 and/or band count >10%% (2 pts) Creatinine 1.5 fold >baseline (2 pts) Abdominal peritoneal signs (3 pts) Vasopressors required (5 pts) Mechanical ventilation attributable to C. Diff (5 pts) Disorientation, confusion, decreased consciousness (5 pts)	1–3 mild to moderate disease 4–6 severe disease 7 or more severe, complicated Retrospectively validated to predict the need for surgery
CARDS [16]	Critical care/ICU admission (5 pts) Age 18–40 (0 pts); 41–60 (2 pts); 61–80 (3 pts); 81–100 (4 pts) Renal failure (acute) (3 pts) Diabetes (−1 pt) Serious comorbidities: Cardiopulmonary (1 pt); liver disease (2 Pts); inflammatory bowel disease (2 pts); malignancy (2 pts)	Score to predict mortality; large derivation and validation cohorts 0 pts mortality 0.33–1.15% 5 pts mortality 4.4–4.5% 10 pts mortality 20.8–23.3% 15 pts mortality 48.1–49.7% 18 pts mortality 100%
ATLAS [17]	Age <60 (0 pts); 60–79 (1 pt); >80 (2 pts) Treatment with systemic antibiotics during CDI therapy (2 pts) Leukocyte count <16 K (0 pts); 16–25 K (1 pt); >25 K (2 pts) Albumin >3.5 (0 pts); 2.6–3.5 (1 pt); <2.5 (2 pts) Serum creatinine <1.57 (0 pts); 1.58–2.35 (1 pt); >2.36 (2 pts)	Patients excluded if presented with WBC > 30, temp > 40, shock or peritonitis. Validated response to predict treatment response and mortality; scores or 3 or less have >85% cure; 4–6 74–81% cure; 7–9 40–62.5% cure
MGH score [18]	Age > 70 (2 pts) WBC >20 or <2 (1 pt) Cardiorespiratory failure (7 pts) Diffuse abdominal tenderness (6 pts)	Value greater than or equal to 6 predicts higher risk patients

Table 14.4 Indications for operative management in patients with *CDI*

A diagnosis of clostridium difficile colitis as determined by one of the following:
1. Positive laboratory assay
2. Endoscopic findings
3. CT scan findings consistent with *c. difficile* colitis (pancolitis +/− ascites)

Plus any one of the following criteria:
1. Peritonitis
2. Perforation
3. Sepsis
4. Intubation
5. Vasopressor requirement after resuscitation
6. Mental status changes
7. Unexplained clinical deterioration
8. Renal failure
9. Lactate >5 mmol/L
10. White blood cell count greater or equal to 50,000 cells/microliter
11. Abdominal compartment syndrome
12. Patients on maximal therapy for complicated CDI that fail to improve within 5–7 days as determined by resolving symptoms and physical exam, and WBC/band count

a vancomycin pulse and taper type of regimen, with an initial course being followed by a progressively decreasing frequency of doses. However, as stated above, second recurrences may be an arena for the use of fidaxomicin. Some clinicians have utilized fidaxomicin pulse and tapers successfully, even in subsequent recurrences, but these are only isolated reports at this point [6].

The therapy that is advocated with third or more recurrences is the use of fecal microbiota therapy [7]. This idea that one could restore normal colonic flora and thus reverse infection and colonization has been present for decades. In recent years, this has truly gained traction, with early work from van Nood et al. demonstrating great success in patients with recurrent disease [8]. Donors have most commonly been family members or known to patients. Resources and research interest have increased for fecal microbiota therapy. There are now sites available to purchase frozen fecal specimens that have been tested for C. difficile and other common pathogens. Additionally, investigations into cultured regimens that represent normal colonic flora are in various stages of investigation and hold the promise for future treatment of the disease. The potential role of fecal microbiota therapy in the treatment of initial or severe disease exists and has been reported, but is not well studied at this point [9].

Minimally Invasive Approaches for the Treatment of CDI

The indications for operative intervention include patients with severe, complicated CDI that are deteriorating despite appropriate nonoperative management and patients with organ dysfunction or sepsis (Table 14.4). Total or subtotal abdominal colectomy has evolved as the operative standard of care, based upon early comparisons versus segmental colectomy. While CDI can be segmental in nature, it is more often a pancolitis. If truly segmental, multiple areas throughout the colon may still be affected. Furthermore, the colon is usually nonischemic, non-perforated, and relatively bland appearing from the serosal surface, making it difficult to determine focal areas of disease for resection.

A total or subtotal colectomy can be performed via minimally invasive techniques; however, this can be difficult in patients with this acute disease process given the dilated, edematous colon, and often accompanying ileus and peritoneal ascites. Several minimally invasive treatments for severe, complicated CDI have been advocated. These are highlighted below.

Loop Ileostomy and Colonic Lavage

As mentioned above, in most cases of CDI undergoing operative management, there is neither colonic ischemia nor perforation. Coupled to the ability of many patients to clinically resolve the infection despite advanced disease, this suggests that resection-based surgery may not be necessary. This led to the hypothesis that a surgical therapy that could decrease bacterial count and toxin may adequately treat CDI and allow for resolution of disease without resection of the colon. This can be done by the creation of a loop ileostomy to divert the fecal stream, performing intraluminal "washout" of the colon, as well as delivering antibiotics into the colon lumen postoperatively. In 2011, we published our initial experience with 43 patients using this operative technique [10]. This procedure resulted in reduced mortality and high colonic preservation as compared to an institutional historic cohort of patients matched by APACHE-II and managed by subtotal colectomy in the time period immediately prior to adopting this method. Our current intraoperative protocol is highlighted in Fig. 14.1. We have now performed this operation in over 100 patients and are currently evaluating outcomes, though preliminary interpretation suggests results are similar to those previously published.

The operation is performed via laparoscopy unless not possible (i.e., significant intra-abdominal adhesions). The operative goal is straightforward: rule out perforation and necrosis and bring the terminal ileum through the abdominal wall for creation of a loop ileostomy as access for intraoperative lavage of the colon (Fig. 14.2). Signs of perforation or ischemia include bilious, purulent, or murky ascites as well as gross discoloration of the colon. Once again, these are rare and not inherent to the pathophysiology of the disease process. Perforation or ischemia likely occurs only in the setting of gross hypovolemia and nonocclusive ischemia or as a con-

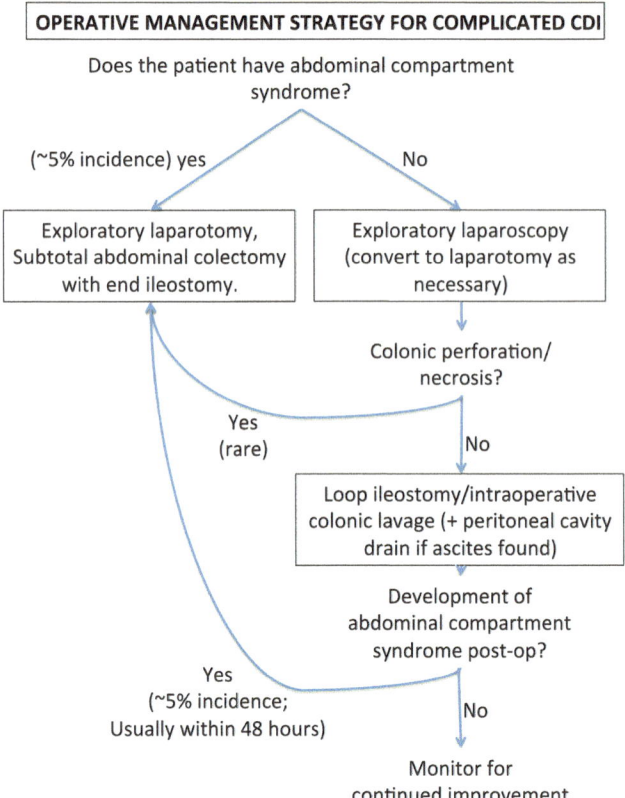

Fig. 14.1 Operative management strategy for complicated CDI

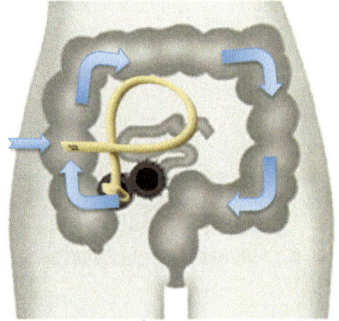

1. Laparoscopic inspection.
2. Bring up ileum for intraoperative lavage of colon and creation of loop ileostomy.
3. Large bore Foley catheter into efferent loop of ileum (balloon below fascia but does not need to be in colon.
4. Lavage with 8 liters of warmed PEG/Balanced Electrolyte solution.
5. Placement of post op Malecot type catheter (~22Fr.) into efferent limp for post-op antegrade vancomycin enemas (500 mg in 500ml LR tid). Secure or put on stopcock to prevent migration into colon.
6. Rectal tube during case and after to facilitate with lavage and enema collection.

Fig. 14.2 Outline of procedure for loop ileostomy and intraoperative colonic lavage for complicated CDI

sequence of the development of abdominal compartment syndrome. A tube is placed through the anal canal preoperatively to help collect the effluent. This can be any formal fecal management system, a rectal tube, or even anesthesia tubing. Placing the patient in lithotomy with a fluid collecting drape system with integrated suction can help to avoid fecal spillage that can occur around whatever tube is used to drain the rectum.

For the intraoperative colonic lavage, we usually utilize a large urinary catheter (26 French) with the balloon placed below the level of the fascia in the efferent limb of the ostomy. It is not necessary for this to go into the colon through the ileocecal valve. One must assure that the loop of ileum that is brought up for the ostomy is not tethered distally to create a potential obstruction during the irrigation. The balloon is usually filled with 10 cc of water. This is enough to prevent backflow without risk of perforating the small intestine. We routinely leave our laparoscopic ports in place and desufflate the abdomen during the irrigation, allowing us the opportunity to quickly inspect the peritoneal cavity at any point during the procedure and at the completion of irrigation. We usually do not mature the ileostomy until the completion of the procedure. The irrigation is performed through a small enterotomy in the terminal ileum with placement of a purse-string suture to hold the urinary catheter in place. However, port sites can be closed and dressed, and the ileostomy can be matured prior to irrigation. In our experience, we have not seen wound infections even with violation of the small bowel prior to wound closure.

We utilize a polyethylene glycol/balanced electrolyte solution (Go-Lytley©) for colonic lavage. It is important to warm the solution to body temperature prior to irrigation to prevent hypothermia. We routinely perform this irrigation with a total of 8 liters. Care must be taken to assure the correct orientation and instillation into the colon and not the proximal small intestine. Effluent can usually be seen exiting the anal tube after the first 1.5–2 liters has been instilled.

A peritoneal drain, which we initially only placed selectively, is now placed in all patients to manage ascites that may develop postoperatively. In patients that presented with acute renal failure and/or ongoing requirement of significant volume resuscitation, the possibility for the development of abdominal compartment syndrome exists; thus, the drain is placed to diminish the potential contribution of ascites to this pathophysiological process.

At the completion of the procedure, a 22 Fr. Malecot tube is left in the efferent limb of the ileostomy below the level of the fascia. Again this does not need to be through the ileocecal valve. We advocate either placement of a three-way stop cock on the end of catheter or a suture secured to a looped red rubber catheter used as an ileostomy bar. These steps are performed to prevent potential peristalsis of the Malecot tube into the colon (which we have seen in two of our patients and verbally communicated to our group from other surgeon experiences). Postoperatively vancomycin enemas are delivered in an anterograde fashion through the Malecot. We uti-

lize a dose of 500 mg three times a day in a volume of 500 mL. This dosing regimen was chosen somewhat arbitrarily and reflects approximately one instillation per shift. Vancomycin enemas are prepared in Ringer's Lactate at our institution, since the standard preparation in normal saline may have contributed to hyperchloremia in three patients.

A difference between loop ileostomy/colonic lavage and subtotal colectomy is that although the procedure can successfully reverse the disease process and reduce bacterial and toxin load, the inflamed colon remains in place and can continue to drive a systemic inflammatory response for several days. Although many patients will show immediate clinical improvement, some will only show a subtle clinical improvement and then plateau for 3–5 days. Serum WBC counts and bandemia may even worsen on postoperative day 1. Colectomy can be performed if patients develop compartment syndrome or continue to clinically deteriorate. CT scan imaging is of limited value as this often reveals continued colonic edema and inflammation for several weeks, even with complete clinical resolution of the disease process.

The absolute contraindications to this approach described include colonic necrosis, perforation, or distal colonic obstruction. Additionally, we advocate performing a subtotal colectomy in any patient with abdominal compartment syndrome preoperatively, given that decompressive laparotomy is necessary. There are no other absolute or relative contraindications, other than that which makes sense based upon coexisting colonic pathology (i.e., associated inflammatory bowel disease). There are no clearly identified patient populations or clinical scenarios otherwise to suggest that colectomy would be indicated in place of loop ileostomy/colonic lavage.

The success of loop ileostomy and colonic lavage is presumably based upon decreasing bacterial counts and levels of toxin. Diversion of the fecal stream and colonic washout may also decrease bacterial translocation and/or systemic endotoxemia in the injured colon. Other factors that may contribute to disease resolution include changing the colonic oxygen concentration and microbiology of the colon as well as possible pharmacologic effects of polyethylene glycol.

Reversal of loop ileostomy can be performed once the patient convalesces from their clinical illness and the underlying associated comorbid diseases allow for a second operation. In our series, this is usually at least 3 months after the initial loop ileostomy and colonic lavage. We do not routinely perform testing for C. difficile prior to reversal of ileostomy. Colonoscopy or contrast-based enemas are performed as indicated to confirm no distal mass lesions or obstructions. Diversion colitis is often found upon colonoscopy. At the time of ileostomy reversal, we advocate a single vancomycin enema through the ileostomy and avoid the use of systemic antibiotics. The ileostomy skin incision is narrowed but not closed completely and packed with wicked ribbon gauze.

Although we have seen low rates of CDI following reversal (5% and all adequately treated with oral vancomycin), others have communicated episodes of acute severe, complicated disease. The addition of fecal microbiota therapy into the ileostomy prior to reversal is being investigated.

Blowhole/Turnbull Ostomy

The creation of a loop ileostomy and blowhole colostomy has been used in patients with "toxic megacolon" for many years. This has most typically been described in pregnant patients with ulcerative colitis; however, multiple reports in patients with CDI have been reported with clinical resolution of the disease. This is a relatively minimally invasive procedure. In the Turnbull or Turnbull-Weakly procedure, a skin level blowhole ostomy of the transverse colon is performed, with a loop ileostomy [11]. This eliminates the need for a major resection.

Others have reported success in the management of severe, complicated CDI with only the creation of a diverting loop colostomy [12]. Similar to loop ileostomy and colonic lavage, if the colon is not perforated or necrotic, the diversion of the fecal stream may be enough to permit resolution of the disease process. This procedure also brings into question the potential benefit of changing intracolonic oxygen tensions that may subsequently alter the microbiology and allow for resolution of CDI. As before, the diseased colon left in place may still drive a persisting inflammatory response.

Vancomycin Enemas/Long Colonic Decompressive Tubes

Intracolonic vancomycin enemas have been utilized as a therapy for CDI for many years. This approach has typically been advocated in the setting of ileus or abdominal distention, where peristalsis and forward flow may not reliably deliver vancomycin into the colon. There is no standard dosing and enema volume, but intuitively it seems that the volume of the enema should be high enough to reflux toward the right colon. Kim et al. described a recent experience with vancomycin enemas using a dose of 1 gm in 500 mL four times a day, in addition to continuing oral vancomycin and intravenous metronidazole, with a high rate of resolution in patients with severe CDI [13]. In addition to the direct delivery of antibiotics, these larger volume enemas may also provide a component of colonic irrigation. Some practitioners have advocated for the adjunctive colonoscopic placement of a long decompressive tube into the right colon followed by essentially antegrade vancomycin enema treatment through the tube [14]. While this may be less invasive than operative intervention, the procedure still requires sedation and carries the inherent risk of perforation from performing a colonoscopy in a distended and diseased colon.

Conclusion

Minimally invasive approaches to the patient with severe, complicated CDI are possible and are an alternative to subtotal colectomy. As experiences continue to evolve, nuanced care for various clinical scenarios may emerge to suggest which therapy may be best for the individual patient. The key for successful surgical management in patients with severe, complicated CDI continues to be early surgical consultation, and appropriate escalation to surgical management prior to major cardiovascular decompensation.

Take-Home Messages: Clostridium difficile colitis leads to considerable morbidity and mortality Proper treatment hinges on appropriate stratification of disease severity Minimally invasive options including loop ileostomy and lavage may help limit morbidity of CDI.

Key References

1. Leffler DA, Lamont JT. Clostridium difficile Infection. N Engl J Med. 2015;372:1539–48.
2. Carter GP, et al. Defining the roles of TcdA and TcdB in localized gastrointestinal disease, systemic organ damage, and the host response during Clostridium difficile infections. MBio. 2015;6:1–10.
3. Lim SK, et al. Emergence of a ribotype 244 strain of clostridium difficile associated with severe disease and related to the epidemic ribotype 027 strain. Clin Infect Dis. 2014;58:1723–30.
4. Surawicz CM, et al. Guidelines for diagnosis, treatment, and prevention of Clostridium difficile infections. Am J Gastroenterol. 2013;108:478–98.
5. Cornely OA, et al. Clinical efficacy of fidaxomicin compared with vancomycin and metronidazole in Clostridium difficile infections: a meta-analysis and indirect treatment comparison. J Antimicrob Chemother. 2014;69:2892–900.
6. Soriano MM, Danziger LH, Gerding DN, Johnson S. Novel Fidaxomicin treatment regimens for patients with multiple Clostridium difficile infection recurrences that are refractory to standard therapies. Open Forum Infect Dis. 2014;1:ofu069.
7. Drekonja D, et al. Fecal microbiota transplantation for Clostridium difficile infection: a systematic review. Ann Intern Med. 2015;162:630–8.

8. van Nood E, et al. Duodenal infusion of donor feces for recurrent *Clostridium difficile*. N Engl J Med. 2013;368:407–15.

9. Waltz P, Zuckerbraun B. Novel therapies for severe Clostridium difficile colitis. Curr Opin Crit Care. 2016;22:167–73.

10. Neal MD, Alverdy JC, Hall DE, Simmons RL, Zuckerbraun BS. Diverting loop ileostomy and colonic lavage. Ann Surg. 2011;254:423–9.

11. Remzi FH, et al. Current indications for blow-hole colostomy:ileostomy procedure. A single center experience. Int J Colorectal Dis. 2003;18:361–4.

12. Oppermann TE, Christopherson WA, Stahlfeld KR. Fulminant Clostridium difficile colitis isolated to the ascending colon by a diverting transverse loop colostomy. Am Surg. 2009;75:859–60.

13. Kim PK, et al. Intracolonic vancomycin for severe *Clostridium difficile* colitis. Surg Infect. 2013;14:532–9.

14. Causey MW, et al. Colonic decompression and direct intraluminal medical therapy for Clostridium difficile-associated megacolon using a tube placed endoscopically in the proximal colon. Color Dis. 2014;16:71–4.

15. Julien M, et al. Severe complicated clostridium difficile infection: can the UPMC proposed scoring system predict the need for surgery? J Trauma Acute Care Surg. 2016; doi:10.1097/TA.0000000000001112.

16. Kassam Z, et al. Clostridium difficile associated risk of death score (CARDS): a novel severity score to predict mortality among hospitalised patients with C. difficile infection. Aliment Pharmacol Ther. 2016;43:725–33.

17. Miller MA, et al. Derivation and validation of a simple clinical bedside score (ATLAS) for Clostridium difficile infection which predicts response to therapy. BMC Infect Dis. 2013;13:148.

18. van der Wilden GM, et al. Fulminant Clostridium difficile colitis: prospective development of a risk scoring system. J Trauma Acute Care Surg. 2014;76:424–30.

Bradley W. Thomas and Ronald F. Sing

Introduction

Abdominal pathology in the intensive care unit (ICU) commonly arises secondary to complications from initial surgery or traumatic injury, missed injury, hypoperfusion (particularly in the setting of vasopressors), or simply as a sequela of long-term severe illness. The critically ill patient often has an unreliable or unobtainable physical exam. Additionally, abdominal sepsis carries a mortality rate of 30–50%, which can be improved by prompt diagnosis [1]. The need for high levels of pulmonary and/or cardiovascular support may create a significant transportation hazard in the critically ill patient. Ultimately, intra-abdominal pathology can be a diagnostic dilemma in the ICU.

Preoperative Diagnostic Options

A multitude of diagnostic studies are widely used as adjuncts to clinical exam and laboratory studies in the critically ill patient. In the absence of pneumoperitoneum, plain film X-rays have limited utility and rarely drive the decision to operate. Ultrasound (US) is effective at evaluating pleural space, cardiac dysfunction, free fluid in the abdomen, and hypovolemia but is limited as a diagnostic tool. In the traumatically injured patient, the sensitivity of US for detection of acalculous cholecystitis is only 30% [2]. Though computed tomography (CT) is an excellent diagnostic modality for intra-abdominal pathology, studies have shown similar limited utility in the critically ill patient: sensitivities are as low as 33–48% for detection of acalculous cholecystitis in the ICU population [3]. Additionally, unlike plain film

B.W. Thomas (✉)
Division of Acute Care Surgery, Department of Surgery, Carolinas Medical Center, Charlotte, NC, USA
e-mail: Bradley.Thomas@carolinashealthcare.org

R.F. Sing
The F.H. "Sammy" Ross Jr Trauma Center, Department of Surgery, Carolinas Medical Center, Charlotte, NC, USA

X-rays and US, CT requires transport that presents a risk for the hemodynamically unstable patient. Diagnostic peritoneal lavage (DPL) is used often to investigate suspected intra-abdominal pathology in patients too unstable for transport; however, DPL has a similar risk profile to diagnostic laparoscopy and does not provide definitive information.

Management

Bedside Diagnostic Laparoscopy (BDL)

Laparoscopy performed at the bedside in the ICU allows visualization of the intraperitoneal structures and therapeutic intervention opportunities with much less morbidity than laparotomy at the bedside [4].

The Agency for Healthcare Research and Quality lists four indications for BDL [3]:

- Unexplained sepsis, systemic inflammatory response syndrome (SIRS), or multiorgan failure
- Unexplained metabolic acidosis
- Abdominal pain with signs of sepsis and no obvious indication for laparotomy
- Increase in abdominal distension in the absence of bowel obstruction

An intra-abdominal source of pathology is found in 43% of patients undergoing BDL for these indications [5]. In one study, the average time to perform a BDL was less than that needed to obtain a CT scan [3].

Bedside diagnostic laparoscopy offers distinct advantages over more conventional adjunctive diagnostic tools. Most significant is the ability to provide definitive diagnosis of intra-abdominal pathology, which may guide decisions regarding further operative treatment or potential end-of-life discussions. Additionally, BDL offers potential therapeutic options at the time of the procedure. BDL also has significant limitations: it is invasive, usually requires chemical paralysis, can exacerbate hypercapnic respiratory failure or worsen preload in a volume-depleted patient, is ineffective for evaluating the retroperitoneum, and requires mobilization of an operating room (OR) team and a laparoscopy tower in most institutions. Patient factors such as previous intra-abdominal surgery with adhesion formation or gaseous distension of the bowel can limit the feasibility of BDL. Despite these limitations, multiple studies have shown a near 100% diagnostic accuracy [3].

Operative Technique

We recommend proceeding with a BDL when the Agency for Healthcare Research and Quality criteria are met. This will provide a definitive diagnosis, obviating the need to transport the critically ill patient to the OR. Standard laparoscopy equipment required to perform a BDL in the ICU includes an insufflator, image processor, light source, cautery, camera head, lens, light cord, trocars, instruments, suture, and monitor (Fig. 15.1). We recommend an experi-

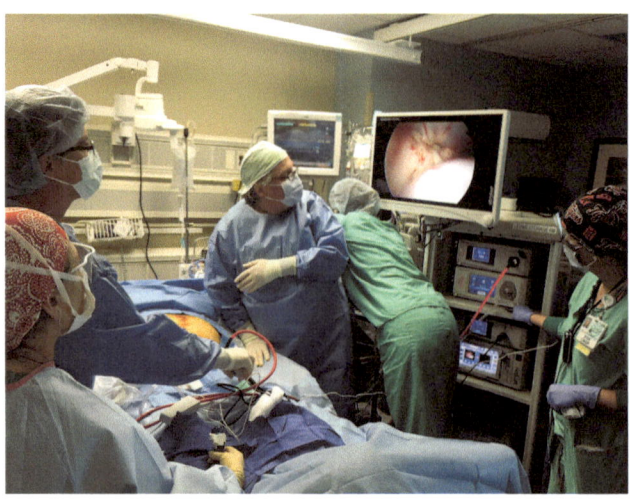

Fig. 15.2 Though space is limited within the intensive care unit compared with the operating room, adequate staff is paramount to perform a bedside diagnostic laparoscopy successfully

enced OR scrub team, nurse, and technician; an individual to serve as an assistant for unexpected needs; an anesthesiologist; and an experienced surgeon (Fig. 15.2). Excellent communication between the surgeon and anesthesiologist is required as the patient is monitored through blood pressure, electrocardiogram, pulse oximetry, and end tidal CO_2 [6]. This monitoring is typical for a critically ill patient. While inhaled anesthetic may be used in the ICU, we recommend total intravenous anesthesia (TIVA) to minimize the equipment that must be transferred from the OR. The surgeon should utilize 5-mm ports and instruments to minimize equipment needs. We prefer the open Hasson technique to access the peritoneal space; however, the method most comfortable for the operating surgeon should be used. Pneumoperitoneum should be limited to 8–10 mmHg pressure, rather than the standard 15 mmHg pressure, to decrease CO_2 absorption, minimize effect on preload, and reduce blood pressure. It is technically feasible to avoid chemical paralytics and perform BDL under local anesthetic and low insufflation pressure. The use of alternative gases such as N_2O, helium, and air has been described with the potential benefit of decreased hypercarbia/acidosis; however, both air and N_2O pose a significant risk of nitrogen or air embolus. In our experience, low pressure (8–10 mmHg) CO_2 is familiar to the OR team, readily available, safe, and does not compromise the ability to successfully visualize the peritoneal cavity; therefore, we use only CO_2. The surgeon is careful to avoid injury to the bowel or cause bleeding. When the procedure is complete, the patient is monitored for any signs of bleeding at additional port sites following removal, and the umbilical port site is closed with a 0 polyglactin suture in a figure-of-eight fashion.

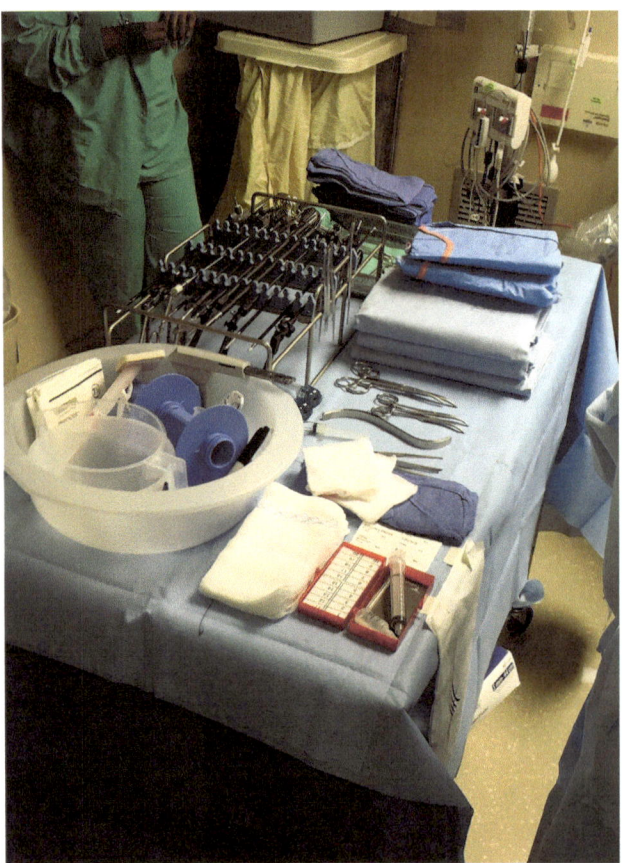

Fig. 15.1 Laparoscopic tower, instrument tray, and scrub tech set up in the intensive care unit

Diagnostic Findings

Bedside diagnostic laparoscopy provides diagnostic information to guide decision making, such as transport of the patient to the OR for a "directed" laparotomy. While many diagnoses are possible, few are common in the critically ill patient.

Intra-abdominal pathology is defined further as *primary*, i.e., the patient is admitted with abdominal sepsis, versus *secondary*, i.e., unrelated to the primary diagnosis. Some examples of primary intra-abdominal pathology include intra-abdominal abscess, perforated viscus (such as perforated peptic ulcer disease), or bowel perforation. Secondary pathology is a common finding in the critically ill population. In Fig. 15.3, a 54-year-old patient had a negative abdominal US, mild elevation of liver transaminases, and a worsening clinical course. The patient was diagnosed through BDL with acute acalculous cholecystitis, which was treated with a laparoscopic-assisted cholecystostomy tube. Mesenteric ischemia is also common in the critically ill patient population. An 80-year-old woman was hypotensive with an elevated lactate and underwent a CT scan (Fig. 15.4).

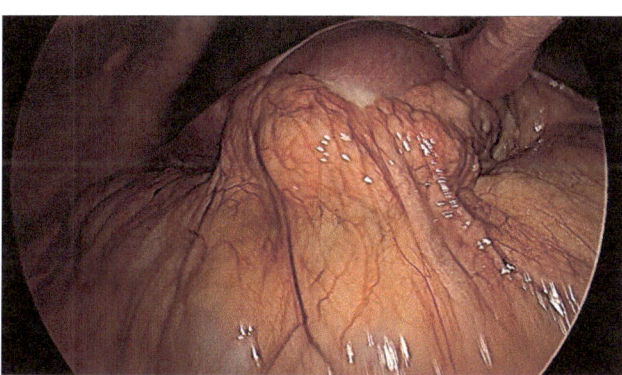

Fig. 15.3 A 54-year-old patient was diagnosed through BDL with acute acalculous cholecystitis

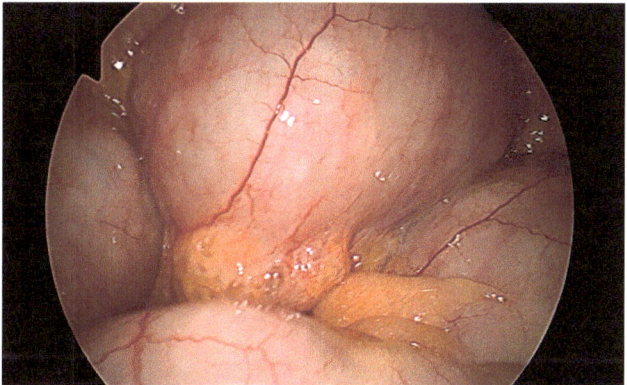

Fig. 15.4 An 80-year-old woman was diagnosed through BDL with pneumatosis intestinalis without signs of necrosis as indicated by computed tomography

A BDL showed clear evidence of pneumatosis intestinalis as indicated by CT but a viable bowel. No further intervention was performed and resuscitation was continued. The patient improved, was extubated, and was discharged from the hospital.

Postoperative Concerns

Complications such as bowel injury, ascitic leak, and bleeding can occur with BDL as with any laparoscopic procedure. We recommend limiting therapeutic interventions during a BDL to simple procedures such as placing a drain or cholecystostomy tube. Done properly BDL is a safe procedure that can significantly aid in definitive diagnosis of intra-abdominal pathology, potentially avoid non-therapeutic laparotomy, and avoid the risk of transport.

Take-Home Messages

1. Intra-abdominal sepsis in the critically ill patient is difficult to diagnose and has a high rate of mortality.
2. Bedside diagnostic laparoscopy (BDL) is a safe, highly diagnostic modality that avoids unnecessary patient transport.
3. BDL should be performed with limited pneumoperitoneum and requires operative experience.
4. Do not stretch the limits of therapeutic intervention at the bedside.

Key References

1. Crandall M, West MA. Evaluation of the abdomen in the critically ill patient: opening the black box. Curr Opin Crit Care. 2006;12(4):333–9.
2. Puc MM, Tran HS, Wry PW, Ross SE. Ultrasound is not a useful screening tool for acute acalculous cholecystitis in critically ill trauma patients. Am Surg. 2002;68(1):65–9.
3. Zemlyak A, Heniford BT, Sing RF. Diagnostic laparoscopy in the intensive care unit. J Intensive Care Med. 2015;30(5):297–302.
4. Diaz JJ Jr, Mauer A, May AK, Miller R, Guy JS, Morris JA Jr. Bedside laparotomy for trauma: are there risks? Surg Infect. 2004;5(1):15–20.
5. Karasakalides A, Triantafillidou S, Anthimidis G, Ganas E, Mihalopoulou E, Lagonidis D, et al. The use of bedside diagnostic laparoscopy in the intensive care unit. J Laparoendosc Adv Surg Tech A. 2009;19(3):333–8.
6. Ceribelli C, Adami EA, Mattia S, Benini B. Bedside diagnostic laparoscopy for critically ill patients: a retrospective study of 62 patients. Surg Endosc. 2012;26(12):3612–5.

Zachary Englert and Jose J. Diaz

Introduction

The modern concept of laparoscopy for trauma began in the 1960s when it was used to detect hemoperitoneum and peritoneal violation for penetrating injuries [1]. The uses for laparoscopy at that time were limited. In the 1980s, laparoscopic surgery became popular, and its indications were expanded again to include the trauma patient. Laparoscopy brought the promise of reduced morbidity associated with negative laparotomies and proved to be a viable therapeutic option for selected injuries in hemodynamically stable patients [2]. Studies have shown time and again that it can be effective in the diagnosis and treatment of both blunt and penetrating abdominal trauma [3–5] leading some to create algorithms to help guide its use and help further define its role in the trauma patient [6, 7].

Diagnostic Tool

Currently, the generally accepted imaging modality for the stable trauma patient is CT scan [8]. However, despite improved diagnostic accuracy, false-negative rates especially for bowel injury remain significant [9]. When unexplained free intraperitoneal fluid is identified on CT scan in a hemodynamically stable patient after trauma, management options include observation, diagnostic peritoneal lavage, diagnostic laparoscopy, and exploratory laparotomy.

The benefits of diagnostic laparoscopy compared to peritoneal lavage or CT include visualization of the source of bleeding as well as the potential for repair of identified injuries [10]. Peritoneal lavage may also be too sensitive of a test. One study reported positive peritoneal lavage lead to a

15–20% nontherapeutic laparotomy rate [11], morbidity that could be avoided if diagnostic laparoscopy were pursued. Despite this, it is unlikely that laparoscopy will completely replace peritoneal lavage or CT for those with a low to moderate index of suspicion, but it can help bridge the gap for these inconclusive screening modalities and reduce the number of nontherapeutic laparotomies.

Laparoscopy for Screening

One of the more common uses for laparoscopy is as a screening tool. It is expected to detect or exclude injury by identifying hemoperitoneum, gastrointestinal spillage, solid organ injury, or peritoneal penetration. A positive finding mandates a formal laparotomy. When compared to traditional screening tools for blunt and penetrating trauma, laparoscopy was shown to be highly sensitive (93–100%) and more specific (80–100%) [12, 13]. It is considered a useful technique in patients who have a moderate or high index of suspicion for intra-abdominal injuries or those who must go to the operating room for non-abdominal procedures. This is the most efficient use of laparoscopy in trauma and is ideal for ruling out peritoneal violation in penetrating injury.

Laparoscopy for Diagnosis

As a diagnostic tool, laparoscopy is expected to detect all injuries that require formal treatment. Unfortunately, complete visualization of the abdominal organs and retroperitoneum can be difficult. Retroperitoneal organs require complex laparoscopic dissection for complete visualization which may be above the skill set for most trauma surgeons. Thus, the results for diagnosis have been less promising; many studies show a missed injury rate of 40% [14–17]. Organs that are traditionally difficult to visualize via laparoscopy such as pancreas, duodenum, and spleen are the most frequently missed. The diagnosis of hollow viscus

Z. Englert (✉) • J.J. Diaz
R Adams Cowley Shock Trauma Center, Program in Trauma,
University of Maryland School of Medicine, Baltimore, MD, USA
e-mail: zacharyenglert@umn.edu; jdiaz@umm.edu

© Springer International Publishing AG 2018
K.A. Khwaja, J.J. Diaz (eds.), *Minimally Invasive Acute Care Surgery*, https://doi.org/10.1007/978-3-319-64723-4_16

injury is also less reliable, with sensitivities of only 18%, but specificities of close to 100% [18]. Consequently, laparoscopy for diagnosis of hollow viscous injury remains controversial. Because of these high rates of missed injuries, a negative laparoscopy should not be taken to mean that occult injuries are absent [19].

Laparoscopy for Treatment

As a therapeutic tool, laparoscopy is expected to definitively repair any injuries that are identified. Repair of a simple diaphragmatic injury from a gunshot or stab wound is ideal and feasible for most surgeons. Although reported less frequently, other injuries that are amenable to laparoscopic repair include cholecystectomy, control of bleeding liver injuries, and closure of a gastrotomy [2]. It also has shown a high success rate for primary repairs to the mesentery and bowel [20]. Some of these repairs may be feasible but are infrequently encountered, and therefore an expertise can be difficult to obtain. Its use to repair bowel injuries without a confirmatory laparotomy is not recommended as standard of care at this time because of the high risk of occult or iatrogenic injuries [19]. Technical success with any repair is dictated by patient selection and specific injury pattern. Therefore, laparoscopy for definitive operative repair must be applied carefully at the discretion of an experienced laparoscopist with extensive experience in the surgical management of trauma.

Patient Selection

Laparoscopy in the trauma population is indicated only in the stable patient and should not be attempted in the face of hemodynamic instability. The unstable patient will not tolerate the time needed to set up essential equipment nor will their physiology endure pneumoperitoneum. For example, a diaphragm injury can cause tension physiology which can lead to hemodynamic collapse in an already unstable patient. In addition, complete visualization of the intra-abdominal structures will be impossible in the face of hemoperitoneum, and this should be considered an indication to convert to an open procedure. There are many relative contraindications to laparoscopy, and these are outlined in Table 16.1 [21]. Specifically, in the setting traumatic brain injury, hypercarbia can have a detrimental effect in brain perfusion and laparoscopy should not be considered in this patient population. In addition, the significance of a prolonged respiratory acidosis due to CO_2 absorption on the injured brain during a laparoscopic procedure has not been studied.

A number of injury patterns, however, can be appropriate for a laparoscopic approach. Patients sustaining low velocity

Table 16.1 Contraindications to laparoscopy in the trauma patient

Absolute	Relative
Hemodynamic instability (SBP < 90 mmHg)	Known intra-abdominal trauma
Hemorrhagic shock	Posterior penetrating trauma
Frank peritonitis	Retroperitoneal injury
Evisceration	Coagulopathy
Traumatic brain injury (GCS < 12)	Acute lung injury
–	Prior abdominal surgery
–	Limited laparoscopic expertise
–	Pregnancy
–	Combined intra- and extra-abdominal injury

Table 16.2 Indications for laparoscopy according to mechanism

Penetrating mechanism	Blunt mechanism
Tangential abdominal wounds	Equivocal CT findings
Flank wounds	Peritonitis
Fascial penetration on local exploration	Unreliable exam secondary to altered mental status
Thoracoabdominal injuries	Strong suspicion for abdominal injury
Positive FAST	–
Peritonitis	–
Equivocal CT findings	–

abdominal or flank gunshot wounds, patients with anterior abdominal stab wounds with fascial penetration, patients sustaining penetrating thoracoabdominal injuries, patients with positive FAST exams, patients with peritonitis, and patients with equivocal abdominal CT scans [10] are all potential candidates. For blunt injury, laparoscopy is appropriate when CT findings are worrisome for hollow viscous injury, when physical examination findings suggest peritonitis, or when physical examination findings are unreliable secondary to altered mental status [10]. Indications for laparoscopy according to mechanism are listed in Table 16.2.

Risks and Benefits

The gold standard exploratory laparotomy is an accurate and effective means of diagnosing and treating abdominal trauma, but it does not come without risk. The general morbidity can be as high as 20–40% with a 3% long-term risk of bowel obstruction [22, 23], making the consequences of a negative laparotomy significant. Laparoscopy has been shown to prevent unnecessary laparotomy in 34% of cases [14–17] and has the benefit of reduced postoperative pain, decreased adhesion formation [24], and decreased length of stay for patients who would have otherwise required a laparotomy. For penetrating trauma, the mean length of stay has been shown to improve by up to 12 days in patients undergoing laparoscopy when compared to those who undergo laparotomy [10]. Similarly, in blunt trauma, laparoscopic approach has shown to decrease the length of stay by approximately 11 days [10]. These figures translate into a lower hospital cost when compared to patients undergoing negative laparotomy [25].

However, like laparotomy, laparoscopy does not come without its own risks. Because of necessary equipment and setup time, definitive treatment can be significantly delayed. The mechanics of laparoscopy can lead to tension pneumothorax, air embolism, bowel injury, intra-abdominal vessel injury, and intracranial hypertension. Carbon dioxide use for pneumoperitoneum has also been shown to cause intracranial hypertension in animal models [26] and should therefore be avoided in patients with suspected head injury.

Procedure

Currently, laparoscopy is most commonly used as a screening modality as part of the initial evaluation of a hemodynamically stable trauma patient. Although there are reports of laparoscopy being performed in the emergency room, the majority of institutions perform the procedure in the operating room where there is optimal access to equipment and better versatility for conversion to open techniques. Various laparoscopic techniques are applicable and subjective preference will drive decisions until experience and reported data increases.

Generally, the patient is placed in the supine position. Arms can be tucked or extended based on the surgeon's preference. Tucked arms will facilitate full range of the surgeon during exploration in both the upper and lower quadrants however will make open exploration more difficult if needed. The patient should be carefully secured to the operating table to ensure stability in full Trendelenburg and reverse Trendelenburg positions. May options are available for abdominal access (Veress needle, Hasson technique, direct trocar insertion) and the operating surgeon should use his/her most comfortable technique. A 10-mm supra- or infraumbilical port is placed and pneumoperitoneum is achieved, maintaining a pressure of 10–15 mm Hg [27]. A 30°, 10-mm laparoscope generally provides the best visualization during exploration. Two 5-mm working ports are then placed in the left and right paramedian sites (Fig. 16.1) [10, 20].

A complete, full, and regimented exploration begins with global inspection of the peritoneal cavity. The abdomen can be open if gross blood or succus is identified. If blood or succus is not identified, the patient is placed in reverse Trendelenburg position to allow for visualization of the upper abdominal organs (liver, spleen, anterior surface of the stomach, omentum, transverse colon, and diaphragm).

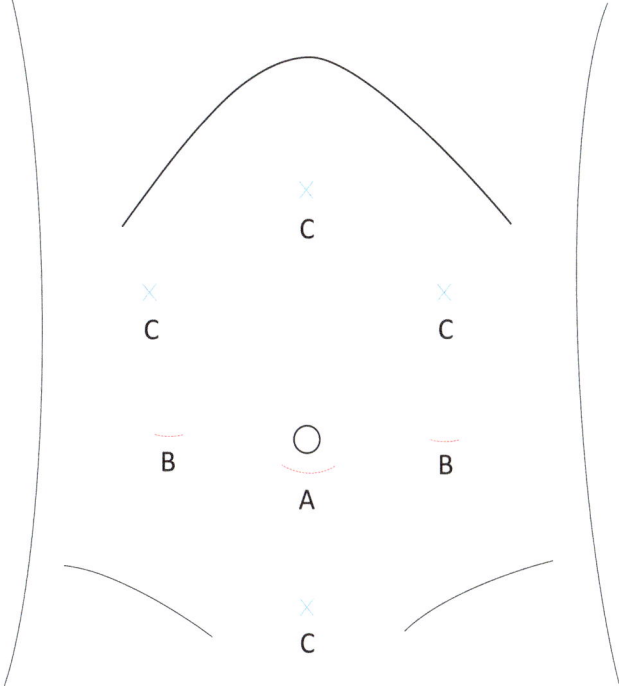

Fig. 16.1 Initial laparoscopic trocar placement for diagnostic laparoscopy. (**a**) 10-mm laparoscope port. 10-mm 30° laparoscope is recommended for optimal visualization. (**b**) 5-mm working ports. (**c**) Options for additional working ports depending on the injury identified

The pancreas and posterior wall of the stomach are accessed by opening the lesser sac via the gastrocolic ligament.

Next, the small bowel is evaluated using a hand-to-hand technique with atraumatic grasping forceps starting at the ligament of Treitz. As the bowel is handed off, the mesentery is inspected for hematoma or penetrating injury. Graspers are rotated 180° in order to inspect the opposite face of the mesentery [27]. The intraperitoneal portion of the colon is manipulated in a similar fashion. Suspicious areas of the retroperitoneum can be better visualized by mobilizing the colon along the peritoneal reflection. The patient can be rotated to better facilitate visualization. Finally, the pelvis is explored by placing the patient in steep Trendelenburg with rotation to the necessary side as needed to evaluate the rectum, bladder, and retroperitoneum.

If significant injury is discovered, additional working ports can be placed in the suprapubic and/or upper quadrants (Fig. 16.1) [20]. If a thoracoabdominal injury is present, the additional ports are placed on the ipsilateral side of the injury. Conversely, if a penetrating wound is isolated to the abdomen, the additional working port typically is placed on the contralateral paramedian location to allow optimal inspection of the anterior abdominal wall for peritoneal penetration [27].

The keys to success in the diagnosis and treatment of traumatic injury with laparoscopy include systematic exploration

Table 16.3 Indications for conversion to open laparotomy

Hemodynamic instability
Duodenal perforation
Periduodenal hematoma
Zone I retroperitoneal hematoma
Zone II/III expanding retroperitoneal hematoma
Intolerance of pneumoperitoneum

[27], appropriate position changes, careful port placement, and technical ability and experience. It is also important for the surgeon to know when to convert to an open procedure. These are outlined in Table 16.3 [20].

Specific Injury Patterns

Injuries to the diaphragm are well suited for laparoscopic diagnosis and treatment. It has a high sensitivity, specificity, and negative predictive value in penetrating trauma. Some authors have had success with observation when these injuries are isolated to the right upper quadrant [28, 29]; however, injuries to the diaphragm in the left upper quadrant should always be repaired to prevent herniation and possible strangulation of viscera. Intracorporeal suturing or laparoscopic suturing devices (Endo Stitch TM) can be used to close the defect in either a figure of eight or horizontal mattress fashion.

Evaluation of the duodenum is more difficult and requires mobilization of the hepatic flexure to adequately inspect the anterior portion of the duodenum and porta hepatis for paraduodenal hematoma or duodenal injury. Mobilization of the second and third portion of the duodenum can be accomplished by a Kocher maneuver to assess the posterior wall and head of the pancreas. These exposures can be difficult and should only be attempted by surgeons skilled in advanced laparoscopy [30].

Treatment of injuries to the small bowel varies based on extent of the injured segment. As a diagnostic tool, laparoscopy has a 40% missed injury rate [15]. Hand-assisted laparoscopic exploration can be more accurate than laparoscopic exploration alone (63 vs 38%) but still has relatively high rates of missed injuries [31]. However, recent reports show that laparoscopic approaches to isolated bowel rupture in blunt trauma offered equivalent results as laparotomy with no difference in postoperative complication and decreased operative blood loss, with only minimally increased mean operative times [32]. It also has the benefit of less adhesion formation [24], less time to recovery, and faster wound healing. When an injury is identified, the bowel is grasped by an atraumatic grasper or Babcock forceps. The umbilical port is removed, and the incision is extended. The bowel is brought out by gentle traction through the umbilical port site. The bowel is inspected manually and repaired or

resected extracorporeal at the discretion of the surgeon. After the repair, the bowel is reinserted back into the abdomen and the port can be replaced [32].

Portions of the solid organs can be directly visualized with the laparoscope. The posterior portions of the liver and spleen however are not easily seen and CT scan should be utilized for more complete information about the presence and nature of these solid organ injuries [30].

The retroperitoneum is classically difficult to examine via laparoscopy. Although, accessibility is expanding because of experience with adrenalectomy, nephrectomy, and colon resection. Currently, laparoscopic retroperitoneal exploration for trauma has yet to be formally described and evidence or concern for injury is an indication for open laparotomy [27].

The use of laparoscopic pericardial window has been described in stable patients with penetrating precordial and thoracoabdominal injuries. In these cases, the pericardium can be accessed and inspected through the central tendon of the diaphragm. If the pericardium appears opaque and does not reflect a bright sheen from the light from the laparoscope, hemopericardium should be suspected. Opening the pericardium under pneumoperitoneum should not be perused if a cardiac injury is suspected because of the potential danger for gas embolism [33]. Experience with this approach is limited and confirmatory open subxiphoid window should be strongly considered with any abnormal findings.

Additional time is required to perform therapeutic procedures on injured organs. It is essential that the patient is physiologically stable and does not have multiple associated injuries. It is important to have quality, up-to-date equipment and instrumentation before attempting organ repair. Hand-assisted techniques may provide better opportunities for exposure and easier specimen removal through greater organ manipulation [34]. As always, the operating surgeon should be familiar and comfortable with hand-assisted laparoscopic surgical principles to properly utilize this technique. Preoperative embolization of injured organs may provide added hemostasis for safer laparoscopic operation.

Complications

Despite the advantages that laparoscopy offers, there are many procedure-related complications that the operating surgeon must be aware and able to immediately and effectively remedy.

Equipment Failure

Although infrequent if equipment is properly maintained, failure in the trauma scenario can produce unacceptable delays in an otherwise life-threatening situation. Examples include damage to the laparoscopic light source, inadequate supply of insufflation gas, faulty camera, or other software-related issues. If problems occur in the midst of the operation, a prompt decision for conversion to an open procedure should be made based on the patient's clinical status and time to remedy the situation. In a hemodynamically stable patient, short delays can be tolerated [35].

Gas Insufflation

Gas insufflation increases intra-abdominal pressure and thereby potentially affects venous return which can in turn cause hemodynamic compromise in an already intravascular depleted trauma patient. Such hemodynamic changes typically include bradycardia and hypotension caused by vagal stimulation secondary to peritoneal stretch [36]. Immediately release of pneumoperitoneum usually corrects the problem. Placement in Trendelenburg position can also help to maximize venous return. If the patient cannot tolerate pneumoperitoneum, the laparoscopic approach should be aborted [35].

Access and Trocar-Related Complications

There are a variety of techniques for accessing the peritoneal cavity (Hasson, Veress needle, direct trocar insertion) all of which are associated with their own specific complications. The intra-abdominal vessels and solid or hollow organs are at risk during abdominal access [37]. Risk factors for access-related complications include obesity, thin body habitus, and anticoagulation. Although rare, the sequela of such injuries (hemorrhage, peritonitis, and multi-organ failure) [37] can be life threatening.

Diaphragm Injury

Injury to the diaphragm is rare, only occurring in 0.4% in a series of 1850 patients undergoing laparoscopic procedures [38]. Injuries typically occur during trocar insertion, liver retraction, or when using electrocautery. Overt injuries can be identified by direct visualization while minor injuries may be suggested by diaphragmatic billowing under decreased pneumoperitoneum. Decreased breath sounds, hypoxia, elevated end-tidal carbon dioxide, and increased airway pressure can be associated with concomitant pneumothorax [38]. Most patients will tolerate a primary laparoscopic diaphragm repair, and chest tubes are usually unnecessary because residual carbon dioxide tends to resolve quickly and spontaneously [39]. Diaphragm injury does however put the patient at risk for tension physiology under pneumoperitoneum, and

if hemodynamic instability is encountered, pneumoperitoneum should be released and immediate chest decompression should be performed [40].

Pneumothorax

Pneumothorax during laparoscopy is typically related to disruption of the diaphragm either from direct injury or tearing of the muscle from high intra-abdominal pressures. Diffusion of gas into the retroperitoneum that tracks into the pleural space can also result in a pneumothorax [41]. Signs of intraoperative pneumothorax include sudden increase in carbon dioxide, decreased lung compliance, and increased inspiratory pressures. The surgeon may also observe bulging diaphragm on the side of the pneumothorax. Pneumothoraces associated with carbon dioxide insufflation usually resolve spontaneously; however, a chest tube should be inserted if the patient develops signs of hemodynamic instability. Proper use of laparoscopic instruments, limiting insufflation pressures to 10 mmHg, and vigilant monitoring of airway pressures will limit the occurrence of pneumothorax during laparoscopy [35].

Vascular Injury

Vascular injuries occur in about 0.3% of all laparoscopic cases [42] and can be the source of hemorrhage from a number of sites. Hemorrhage at the port site usually occurs during placement of secondary trocars. It is important for trocars to be placed in the midline or away from the epigastric artery to avoid injury. Bleeding may not be apparent because the trocar will provide local tamponade, and therefore removal under direct visualization is important to rule out injury. Major intra-abdominal vessel injury is associated with 15% mortality [43]. The most commonly injured vessels include the common iliac vein, omental vessels, inferior vena cava, and aorta [44]. The vast majority of these injuries occur during initial peritoneal access. In the case of major vascular injury, prompt conversion to an open procedure for primary or prosthetic repair is indicated.

Visceral Injury

During abdominal access and port placement or with the use of electrocautery, the small bowel is at risk of injury with an incidence of up to 0.5% [45]. If these injuries go unnoticed during surgery, the result can be of significant morbidity or mortality. To decrease the chance of bowel or solid organ injury, abdominal entry should take place in a quadrant away from prior surgical scars. While entry technique does not appear to significantly affect injury rate, trocar-associated morbidity from visceral injuries is significantly lower for blunt compared to bladed trocars [46].

Bladder injuries most often occur during suprapubic port placement. The risk of bladder injury can be minimized by preoperative Foley catheter placement. Minor bladder injuries can be managed with primary repair and Foley catheter drainage; more extensive injuries require formal bladder repair which may require laparotomy [47].

Conclusion

Laparoscopy is a safe and effective modality for diagnostic evaluation and management of blunt and penetrating traumatic injuries in select individuals; however, it has yet proven itself successful to be considered standard of care. Those considering this approach should have extensive laparoscopic experience, be aware of technical limitations, be comfortable managing complications, and be proficient in treating injuries by laparotomy. As experience with laparoscopy in trauma increases, the indications will expand and more standardized methods can be developed.

Take-Home Messages

1. The surgeon must make sure the patient is hemodynamically stable and will tolerate a positive pressure pneumoperitoneum.
2. Laparoscopic for trauma is an excellent screening tool for violation of the peritoneum for penetrating injury.
3. The surgeon should be very aware of their individual technical limitations. Most trauma surgeons have limited advance laparoscopic skills. A laparoscopic surgeon may be able to fully evaluate the abdomen. Both must be able to identify an injury with 100% certainty 100% of the time.

Key References

1. Heselson J. The value of Peritoneoscopy as a diagnostic aid in abdominal conditions. Cent Afr J Med. 1963;9:395–8.
2. Zantut L, Ivatury R, Smith R, et al. Diagnostic and therapeutic laparoscopy for penetrating abdominal trauma – a multicenter experience. J Trauma. 1993;42:825–9.
3. Lin H, Wu J, Tu C, Chen H, Shih H. Value of diagnostic and therapeutic laparoscopy for abdominal stab wounds. World J Surg. 2010;34:1653–62.
4. Shah S, Shah K, Joshi P, Somani R, Gohil V, Dakhda S. To study the incidence of organ damage and post-operative care in patients

of blunt abdominal trauma with Haemoperitoneum managed by laparoscopy. J Minim Access Surg. 2011;7:169–72.
5. Marwan A, Harmon C, Georgeson K, Smith G, Muensterer O. Use of laparoscopy in the management of pediatric abdominal trauma. J Trauma. 2010;69:761–4.
6. Hallfeldt K, Trupka A, Erhard J, Waldner H, Schweiberer L. Emergency laparoscopy for abdominal stab wounds. Surg Endosc. 1998;12:907–10.
7. Smith R, Fry W, Morabito D, Koehler R, Organ C. Therapeutic laparoscopy in trauma. Am J Surg. 1995;170:632–6.
8. Brownstein M, Bunting T, Meyer A, Fakhry S. Diagnosis and management of blunt small bowel injury: a survey of the membership of the American Association for the Surgery of Trauma. J Trauma. 2000;48:402–7.
9. Killeen K, Shanmuganathan K, Poletti P, Cooper C, Mirvis S. Helical computed tomography of bowel and mesenteric injuries. J Trauma. 2001;51:26–36.
10. Johnson J, Garwe T, Raines A, Thurman J, Carter S, Bender J, et al. The use of laparoscopy in the diagnosis and treatment of blunt and penetrating abdominal injuries: 10-year experience at a level 1 trauma center. Am J Surg. 2013;205:317–21.
11. Wood D, Berci G, Morgenstern L, et al. Mini-laparoscopy in blunt abdominal trauma. Surg Endosc. 1998;2:184–9.
12. Cuschieri A, Hennessy T, Stephens R, Berci G. Diagnosis of significant abdominal trauma after road traffic accidents: preliminary results of a multicentre clinical trial comparing minilaparoscopy with peritoneal lavage. Ann R Coll Surg Engl. 1988;70:153–5.
13. Lalvino C, Esposito T, Marshall W, et al. The role of diagnostic laparoscopy in the management of trauma patients: a preliminary assessment. J Trauma. 1993;34:506–15.
14. Brandt C, Priebe P, Jacobs D. Potential of laparoscopy to reduce nontherapeutic trauma laparotomies. Am Surg. 1994;60:416–20.
15. Rossi P, Mullins D, Thal E. Role of laparoscopy in the evaluation of abdominal trauma. Am J Surg. 1993;166:707–11.
16. Ortega A, Tang E, Froes E, et al. Laparoscopic evaluation of penetrating thoracoabdominal traumatic injuries. Surg Endosc. 1996;10:19–22.
17. Mazuski J, Shapiro M, Kaminski D, et al. Diagnostic laparoscopy for evaluation of penetrating abdominal trauma. J Trauma. 1997;7:163.
18. Ivantury R, Simon R, Stahl W. A critical evaluation of laparoscopy in penetrating abdominal trauma. J Trauma. 1993;34:822–7.
19. Villavicencio R, Aucar J. Analysis of laparoscopy in trauma. J Am Coll Surg. 1999;189:11–20.
20. Lee P, Chiao L, Wu J, Lin K, Lin H, Ko W. Laparoscopy decreases the laparotomy rate in hemodynamically stable patients with blunt abdominal trauma. Surg Innov. 2014;21:155–65.
21. Guidelines for Diagnostic Laparoscopy. n.d. http://www.sages.org/publications/guidelines/guidelines-for-diagnostic-laparoscopy/. Retrieved May 28, 2016, from Society of American Gastrointestinal and Endoscopic Surgeons.
22. Shih H, Wen Y, Ko T, Wu J, Su C, Lee C. Noninvasive evaluation of blunt abdominal trauma: prospective study using diagnostic algorithms to minimize nontherapeutic laparotomy. World J Surg. 1999;23:265–9.
23. Henderson V, Organ C, Smith R. Negative Trauma Celiotomy. Am Surg. 1993;59:365–70.
24. Schippers E, Tittel A, Ottinger A, Schumpelick V. Laparoscopy vs laparotomy: comparison of adhesions formation after bowel resection in a canine model. Dig Surg. 1998;15:145–7.
25. Marks J, Youngelman D, Berk T. Cost analysis of diagnostic laparoscopy versus laparotomy in the evaluation of penetrating abdominal trauma. Surg Endosc. 1997;11:272–6.
26. Josephs L, Este-McDonald J, Birkett D, Hirsch E. Diagnostic laparoscopy increases intracranial pressure. J Trauma. 1994;36:815–8.

27. Kawahara N, Alster C, Fujimura I, Poggetti R, Birolini D. Standard examination system for laparoscopy in penetrating abdominal trauma. J Trauma. 2009;67:589–95.

28. Carneval N, Baron N, Delany H. Peritoneoscopy as an aid to diagnosis of abdominal trauma: a preliminary report. J Trauma. 1977;17:634–41.

29. Ditmars M, Bongard F. Laparoscopy for triage of penetrating trauma: the decision to explore. J Laparoendosc Surg. 1996;6:285–91.

30. Ransom K, Smith, R. Laparoscopy for trauma. 3rd ed. Paul Alan Wetter M, editor. 2012. http://laparoscopy.blogs.com/prevention_management_3/2011/01/laparoscopy-for-trauma.html. Retrieved May 16, 2016, from Prevention and Management of Laparoendoscopic Surgical Complications.

31. Ashbun H, Bowyer M, Knolmayer T, Wiedeman J. Hand assisted laparoscopic exploration for trauma: a false sense of security. Surg Endosc. 1998;12:614.

32. Omori H, Asahi H, Inoue Y, et al. Selective application of laparoscopic intervention in the management of isolated bowel rupture in blunt abdominal trauma. J Laparoendosc Adv Surg Tech A. 2003;13:83–8.

33. Grewal H, Ivanturi RR, Divakar M, Simon RJ, Rohman M. Evaluation of subxiphoid pericardial window used in the detection of occult cardiac injury. Injury. 1995;26:305–10.

34. Choi Y, Lim K. Therapeutic laparoscopy for abdominal trauma. Surg Endosc. 2003;17:421–7.

35. Kindel T, Latchana N, Swaroop M, Chaudhry U, Noria S, Choron R, et al. Laparoscopy in trauma: an overview of complications and related topics. Int J Crit Illn Inj Sci. 2015;5:196–205.

36. Motew M, Ivankovich A, Bieniarz J, Albrecht R, Zahed B, Scommegna A. Cardiovascular effects and acid-base and blood gas changes during laparoscopy. Am J Obstet Gynecol. 1973;115:1002–12.

37. Bhoyrul S, Vierra M, Nezhat R, Krummel T, Way L. Trocar injuries in laparoscopic Surger. J Am Coll Surg. 2001;192:677–83.

38. Aron M, Colombo J, Turna B, Stein R, Haber G, Gill I. Diaphragmatic repair and/or reconstruction during upper abdominal urologic laparoscopy. J Urol. 2007;169:41–4.

39. Voyles C, Madden B. The "floppy diaphragm" sign with laparoscopic-associated pneumothorax. JSLS. 1998;2:71–3.

40. Goettler CE, Bard MR, Toschlog EA. Laparoscopy in trauma. Curr Surg. 2004;61:554–9.

41. Hawasli A. Spontaneous resolution of massive laparosopy-associated pneumothorax: the case of the bulging diaphragm and review of the literature. J Laparoendosc Adv Surg Tech A. 2002;12:77–82.

42. Jansen F, Kolkman W, Bakkum E, deKroon C, Trimbos-Kemper T, Trimbos J. Complications of laparoscopy: an inquiry about closed versus open entry technique. Am J Obstet Gynecol. 2004;190:634–8.

43. Krishnakumar S, Tambe P. Entry complications in laparoscopic surgery. J Gynecol Endosc Surg. 2009;1:4–11.

44. Pemberton R, Tolley D, van Velthoven R. Prevention and management of complications in urological laparoscopic port site placement. Eur Urol. 2006;50:958–68.

45. Rabl C, Palazzo F, Aoki H, Campos G. Initial laparoscopic access using an optical trocar without pneumoperitoneum is safe and effective in the morbidly obese. Surg Innov. 2008;15:126–31.

46. Antoniou S, Antoniou G, Koch O, Pointner R, Granderath F. Blunt versus bladed trocars in laparoscopic surgery: a systematic review and meta-analysis of randomized trials. Surg Endosc. 2013;27:2312–20.

47. Meyer A, Blanc P, Balique J, Kitamura M, Juan R, Delacoste F, et al. Laparoscopic totally extraperitoneal inguinal hernia repair: twenty-seven serious complications after 4565 consecutive operations. Rev Col Bras Cir. 2013;40:32–6.

Index

A

Abscess, 90
AC. *See* Acute cholecystitis (AC)
ACS. *See* Acute care surgery (ACS)
Acute care surgery (ACS), 46, 47, 49–51
    pneumoperitoneum, 1, 3, 4
Acute cholecystitis (AC), 47
    acalculous cholecystitis, 46
    cholecystectomy (*see* Cholecystectomy)
    complication, 45
    critical view, safety, 48, 50
    CT imaging, 46
    diagnostic assessment, 46
    gallbladder management, 50–51
    inflammation, gallbladder, 45
    jaundice, 46
    postoperative concerns, 49, 50
    pregnant patients, 46
    septic shock, 46
    severity, 45, 46
Acute pancreatitis, 67
    complications, 71–75
    definition, 67, 68
    interventions, 68–71
    laparoscopy/VARD, 69–71
    management, 74
    maximally invasive methods, 68
    minimally invasive methods, 68, 69
    percutaneous drainage, 69
Adjustable gastric banding, 41
Alvarado score, 82
American College of Gastroenterology (ACG), 107
Anastomotic leak
    colorectal anastomosis, 97
    diagnosis, 98
    Hasson technique, 99
    laparoscopic evaluation, 99
    management, 98, 99
    repairing, 99
Antibiotic therapy, 64
Appendicitis
    abdominal emergency, 81
    intraluminal pressure, 81
    lymphoid pulp, 81
    operative technique, 83–86
    patient positioning, 83
    perforated appendicitis, 87
    postoperative concerns, 86, 87
    preoperative diagnostic options, 81, 82
    transection, 86
    uncomplicated appendicitis, 82, 83
    vermiform, 81
Appendicolith, 81, 82
Atlanta Symposium, 67
Atraumatic grasper, 85

B

Bariatric surgery
    BPD-DS, 33
    classification, 33
    gastric bypass (*see* Gastric bypass)
    gastrointestinal leaks, 35–38
    gastrointestinal obstruction, 38
    intraoperative decisions, 35
    laparoscopic suturing, 33
    marginal ulceration, 41–43
    operative complications, 33, 35
    port placement, 35
    Roux-en-Y gastric bypass, 33
    sleeve gastrectomy, 40, 41
    weight loss, 33, 35
BDIs. *See* Bile duct injuries (BDIs)
Bedside diagnostic laparoscopy (BDL)
    complications, 115
    diagnostic findings, 117
    diagnostic laparoscopy, 115
    operative technique, 116, 117
    postoperative concerns, 117
    preoperative diagnostic options, 115
    visualization, 115
Bezoar obstruction, 78–79
Bile duct injuries (BDIs), 47–51
Biliopancreatic diversion with duodenal switch
    (BPD-DS), 33
Blowhole ostomy, 112
BPD-DS. *See* Biliopancreatic diversion with duodenal switch
    (BPD-DS)

C

Cholecystectomy
    acute inflammation, 47
    awareness, gallbladder's inflammation, 47
    BDIs, 47–49
    bile duct time-out, 48, 49
    cognitive maps, 48
    emergency, 47
    injury avoidance, 47, 48
    open surgery and mortality, 47
    port/trocar placement, 47
    postoperative complications, 47
    prophylaxis, 47
    randomized trials, 47, 48

© Springer International Publishing AG 2018
K.A. Khwaja, J.J. Diaz (eds.), *Minimally Invasive Acute Care Surgery*, https://doi.org/10.1007/978-3-319-64723-4

Choledocholithiasis, 55–59
    acute obstruction, 54
    biliary tract disease, 53
    bilirubin stones, 53
    Charcot's triad, 54
    cholesterol, 53
    clinical scenarios and therapeutic options, 55
    diagnosis, 54, 55
    ERCP (see Endoscopic retrograde cholangiopancreatography (ERCP))
    LCBDE (see Laparoscopic common bile duct exploration (LCBDE))
    management, 55
    operative therapy, 56
    pharmacologic prophylaxis, 54
    prevalence, gallstones, 53
    prevention, 54
    Roux-en-Y gastric bypass, 53, 54, 59
    weight loss, 53
Clostridium difficile infection (CDI)
    BI/NAP1/ ribotype 027, 107
    colonic lavage, 110–112
    disease severity, 107–109
    loop ileostomy, 110–112
    medical therapy, 107–109
    pathophysiology, 107
    scoring systems, 109
    severity scoring system, 108
    signs/symptoms, 108
    spore-forming bacillus, 107
Colon
    diverticular disease, 89
    processes, 89
Colonic fistulae, 72
Colonic lavage, 110–112
Colorectal surgery
    anastomotic leak, 97–99
    rectal stump leak, 99–101
    surgical complications, 97
Common bile duct exploration. See Laparoscopic common bile duct exploration (LCBDE)
Computed tomography (CT), 82
Contrast-enhanced computed tomography (CECT), 68
C-reactive protein (CRP) level, 82

D
Diaphragm injury, 123
Diverticulitis
    clinical presentation, 90, 91
    colonic diverticular disease, 89
    elective resection, 91–95
    epidemiology, 89
    operative technique, 92–95
    pathophysiology, 89
Diverticulosis
    and diverticulitis, 89
    mucosa and submucosa, 89
    pneumaturia, 91
    sigmoid, 89

E
Endo Catch bag, 86
Endoscopic retrograde cholangiopancreatography (ERCP), 54, 55, 58, 59
Enhanced recovery after surgery (ERAS), 98
ERCP. See Endoscopic retrograde cholangiopancreatography (ERCP)

F
Fecal microbiota therapy, 109, 112
Fistula, 91
Food bolus, 78–79

G
Gallstone ileus, 79
Gas insufflation, 123
Gastric bypass, 79
    adhesions, 40
    closed-loop obstructions, 38
    gastrojejunal anastomotic strictures, 38
    internal hernia, 38–40
    laparotomy, 38
    Roux limb, 38
    small bowel obstruction, 40
Gastrointestinal hemorrhage, 91
Gastrointestinal leaks
    description, 35
    diagnosis, 36
    management, 36, 37
    postoperative care, 37, 38
Grade B leaks, 98

H
Hand-assisted laparoscopic surgery (HALS), 92
Hartmann's procedure, 94
Hernias, 78
Hiatal hernia, 25, 28, 29
Hinchey classification, 90, 93

I
Ileal pouch-anal anastomosis (IPAA)
    diagnosis, 102
    management, 102, 103
Incarcerated abdominal wall hernias, 15
    blood work, 16
    imaging, 16
    incidence, 15
    inguinal hernias (see Inguinal hernias)
    laboratory workup, 16
    postoperative care, 21, 22
    risk factors, 15
    ventral hernias, 15, 19–21
Infected pancreatic necrosis, 67
Inguinal hernias
    asymptomatic, 15
    incidence, 15
    laparoscopic approach, 16, 17
    operating room, 16
    operative approach, 17–19
    risk factors, 15
    small bowel obstruction, 16
    TAPP, 16–19
Injury patterns, 122
Intensive care unit (ICU)l, 115
Interval appendectomy, 87
Intra-abdominal pathology, 115, 117
Intracolonic vancomycin enemas, 112
Intra-operative cholangiogram (IOC), 56, 57
IOC. See Intra-operative cholangiogram (IOC)

L

Laparoscopic appendectomy, 83–86
Laparoscopic common bile duct exploration (LCBDE)
    choledochotomy, 57, 58
    gastrotomy and intra-operative ERCP, 58, 59
    IOC, 56, 57
    trancystic and trancholecystic approach, 57, 58
Laparoscopic exploration, free air
    access, 9
    adjuncts, 7, 10
    benefits, 12
    C0₂ embolism, 12
    contraindications, 11
    conversion, 10
    equipment, 9
    hemodynamic instability, 11
    indications, 11
    intra-abdominal adhesions, 7
    laparotomy, 7, 10
    methylene blue, 7, 10
    morbidity, 7
    operating room setup, 8
    ower abdomen, 10
    patient positioning, 8, 9
    pneumoperitoneum, 7, 11, 12
    preparation, 7–8
    risks, 11, 12
    steps, 9–10
    upper abdomen, 10
Laparoscopy
    conversion, 92
    initial operative technique, 90
Loop ileostomy, 99, 110–112

M

Marginal ulceration
    diagnosis, 41, 42
    incidence, 41
    management, 42, 43
    postoperative care, 43
Mediastinoscopes, 69
Minimally invasive approach, 91
    goals, 94
    incarcerated abdominal wall hernias, 15–22
    laparoscopic approach, 94
Minimally invasive surgery (MIS)
    ACS, 1
    choledocholithiasis, 53–59
    laparoscopy, pneumoperitoneum, 1–4
    trauma and physiologic stress, 1

N

Nasogastric tube, 64
Necrosectomy, 68, 69, 71
Nephroscopes, 69
Nonsteroidal anti-inflammatory drugs (NSAIDS), 97

P

Pandora's box, 67
PANTER trial, 69
Paraesophageal hernia (PEH)
    acute incarceration, 25, 26
    anti-reflux procedure, 30

    blunt dissection, 28
    capnothorax, 29
    chest radiography, 26
    Collis gastroplasty, 29, 30
    diaphragmatic closure, 30
    endoscopy, 26
    esophagus, 28, 29
    Ethibond sutures, 30
    feeding access, 30, 31
    gastrohepatic ligament, 28
    hiatal hernia, 25, 28, 29
    hypotension, 29
    incidental *vs.* acute, 25, 26
    laboratory tests, 26
    laparoscopic surgery, 27
    manometry, 26
    perforations/ischemic tissue, 28
    permanent/biologic mesh, 30
    physical examination, 26
    postoperative concerns, 31–32
    preoperative preparation, 26–31
    procedure completion, 31
    strangulation, 25, 26, 30
    trocar position, 28
    upper gastrointestinal (UGI), 31
    vagus nerves, 28
    Veress needle, 28
PEH. *See* Paraesophageal hernia (PEH)
Pelvic sepsis, 100
Perforated appendicitis, 87
Perforated ulcers
    abdominal CT scan, 62
    antibiotic Therapy, 64
    blood work, 61
    chest/abdominal X-ray, 61
    complications, 65
    development, 61
    differential diagnosis, 61
    emergency department, 62
    follow Uup, 64
    Helicobacter Pylori eradication, 64
    instruments
        access and exploration, 62
        conversion, 64
        graham patch repair, 63
        omental patch repair, 63, 64
        perforations, 63
        positioning, 62
        repair and closure, 63, 64
    leak and infections, 65
    nasogastric tube and feeding, 64
    peptic ulcer disease, 61
    post-operative care, 64
    surgery *vs.* observation, 62
Perforation, 90
Pneumoperitoneum
    ACS, 3, 4
    cardiac arrhythmias, 3
    cardiac output, 2, 3
    cardiovascular system, 2
    CO₂ insufflation, 1–3
    elevated abdominal pressure, 4
    emergency general surgery, 4
    hypercarbia, 3
    inflammatory markers, 3
    inflammatory response, 3

Pneumoperitoneum (*cont.*)
    neurohumoral factors, 3
    oliguria, 3
    physiologic changes, 1, 2
    renal blood flow, 3
    respiratory changes, 1, 2
    venous gas embolism, 3
Pneumothorax, 3, 123
Prothrombin complex concentrates (PCC), 91

R
Rectal stump leak
    diagnosis, 100
    management, 100, 101
Resuscitative Balloon Occlusion of the Aorta (REBOA), 71
Roux-en-Y gastric bypass, 53, 54, 59

S
Screening, 119
Sepsis, 94
Sequential compression devices (SCDs), 92
Single Incision Laparoscopic Surgery (SILS), 71
Sleeve gastrectomy, 40, 41
Small bowel obstructions
    adhesions, 78
    bezoar obstruction, 78–79
    complications, 79–80
    definition, 77
    diagnosis, 79
    etiology, 77
    food bolus, 78–79
    foreign bodies, 79
    gastric bypass, 79
    hernias, 78
    laparoscopic exploration, 77, 78
    patient selection, 77
    postoperative, 79
    tumors, 79
Supportive care, 67

T
TAPP. *See* Transabdominal preperitoneal (TAPP)
Total intravenous anesthesia (TIVA), 116
Transabdominal preperitoneal (TAPP), 16–19
Trauma
    diagnosis, 119, 120
    diaphragm injury, 123
    equipment failure, 122–123
    laparoscopy, 119
    patient selection, 120
    procedure, 121, 122
    risks and benefits, 120, 121
    screening, 119
    treatment, 120
Trocar placement, 93
Trocar-Related Complications, 123
Tumors, 79
Turnbull ostomy, 112

U
Uncomplicated appendicitis, 82, 83

V
Vancomycin enema, 112
    anterograde fashion, 111
    ileostomy, 111
    treatment of patients, 108
Vascular injuries, 123
Video-assisted retroperitoneal debridement (VARD), 69–71
    completion, 71
    necrotic tissue, 73
    operative steps, 72
    outcomes, 70
Visceral injury, 123–124
Volvulus, 97, 99, 101

W
Walled-off pancreatic necrosis (WOPN), 67